# Disinfection in Healthcare

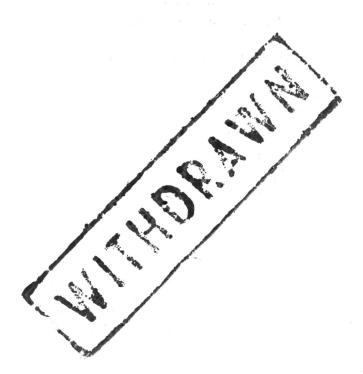

# Disinfection in Healthcare

## 3RD EDITION

### Peter Hoffman
*Clinical Scientist*
*Laboratory of Healthcare-Associated Infection*
*Health Protection Agency*
*London*

### Christina Bradley
*Laboratory Manager*
*Hospital Infection Research Laboratory*
*City Hospital*
*Birmingham*

AND

### Graham Ayliffe
*Emeritus Professor of Medical Microbiology*
*University of Birmingham and Formerly Hon. Director*
*Hospital Infection Research Laboratory*
*City Hospital*
*Birmingham*

**Blackwell**
Publishing

© 2004 Health Protection Agency
Published by Blackwell Publishing Ltd
Blackwell Publishing, Inc., 350 Main Street, Malden, Massachusetts 02148-5020, USA
Blackwell Publishing Ltd, 9600 Garsington Road, Oxford OX4 2DQ, UK
Blackwell Publishing Asia Pty Ltd, 550 Swanston Street, Carlton, Victoria 3053, Australia

The right of the Author to be identified as the Author of this Work has been asserted in accordance with the Copyright, Designs and Patents Act 1988.

First published 1984
(Published by Public Health Laboratory Service)
Second edition 1993
(Published by Public Health Laboratory Service)
Third edition 2004

Library of Congress Cataloging-in-Publication Data

Hoffman, P. N.
    Disinfection in healthcare / by Peter Hoffman, Christina Bradley, and Graham Ayliffe. —3rd ed.
        p. ; cm.
    Rev. ed. of: Chemical disinfection in hospitals / G.A.J. Ayliffe, D. Coates, P.N. Hoffman. 2nd ed. 1993.
    Includes bibliographical references and index.
    ISBN 1-4051-2642-6
    1. Disinfection and disinfectants. 2. Health facilities—Disinfection.
3. Hospitals—Disinfection.
    [DNLM: 1. Cross Infection—prevention & control. 2. Disinfectants—therapeutic use.
3. Disinfection—methods. WX 167 H699d 2004] I. Bradley, Tina. II. Ayliffe, G. A. J.
III. Ayliffe, G. A. J. Chemical disinfection in hospitals. IV. Health Protection Agency
(Great Britain) V. Title.

    RA761.H64 2004
    614.4'8—dc22

                                                            2004007844
ISBN 1-4051-26426

A catalogue record for this title is available from the British Library

Set in 9/12pt Palatino by TechBooks Electronic Services Pvt. Ltd., New Delhi, India
Printed and bound in India by Replika Press Pvt. Ltd.

Commissioning Editor: Maria Khan
Editorial Assistant: Claire Bonnett
Development Editor: Katrina Chandler

For further information on Blackwell Publishing, visit our website:
http://www.blackwellpublishing.com

The publisher's policy is to use permanent paper from mills that operate a sustainable forestry policy, and which has been manufactured from pulp processed using acid-free and elementary chlorine-free practices. Furthermore, the publisher ensures that the text paper and cover board used have met acceptable environmental accreditation standards.

# Contents

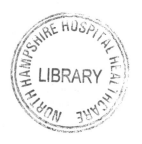

Preface, vii

1 Principles of disinfection, 1

2 Properties of chemical disinfectants, 8

3 Disinfection policy, 17

4 Thermal disinfection, 21

5 Organisms of special significance, 26

6 Cleaning and disinfection of the environment, 40

7 Disinfection of the skin and mucous membranes, 49

8 Disinfection of medical equipment, 64

9 Disinfectants in pathology departments, 73

10 Safety in chemical disinfection, 80

11 Disinfectant testing, 87

Appendix: Summary of policy for decontamination of equipment or environment, 93

Bibliography, 99

Index, 101

# Preface

This book continues a series of publications, the most recent of which was *Chemical Disinfection in Hospitals* by Graham Ayliffe, David Coates and Peter Hoffman in 1993, itself an update of a 1984 edition. The principles of disinfection have changed little since the publication that gave rise to this series (*The use of chemical disinfectants in hospitals*, a Public Health Laboratory Service monograph) written by J C Kelsey and Isobel M Maurer in 1972.

Previous editions were concerned solely with chemical disinfection. We have now included thermal disinfection which, when applied in the controlled conditions of a thermal washer-disinfector, can provide cleaning and disinfection of high quality assurance. We also reflect the increased role of chemical washer-disinfectors, particularly in the decontamination of flexible endoscopes. Both types of washer-disinfector require new testing methods and audit of the departments in which they are used.

The emergence of the prion disease variant Creutzfeldt–Jakob disease (vCJD) since the last edition has had a considerable impact on the whole process of cleaning and disinfection of instruments. The increasing prominence of antibiotic-resistant bacteria, such as methicillin-resistant *Staphylococcus aureus* (MRSA), vancomycin-resistant enterococci and multiply-resistant acinetobacters, demonstrates the need for good cleaning in addition to effective disinfection as part of an integrated infection control approach.

Hands as vectors of infection have long made them of interest in infection control. Alcoholic solutions have been used for many years in some European countries for hand disinfection (hygienic hand disinfection) and are now increasingly used in the UK, the USA and other countries. Alcohol hand disinfection provides an alternative to washing with soap or detergent–disinfectant products, an approach which is having a favourable clinical impact.

Safety aspects of the use of disinfectants impact directly on the use of chemical disinfectants, both in the legal framework and in the application of the law. Respiratory sensitizers such as glutaraldehyde are now being replaced with agents that are safer to use but that can be more damaging to the instruments being decontaminated. They also have to be compatible with the chemical washer-disinfectors now in routine use.

European and national guidelines and legislation on health and safety and decontamination of medical equipment continue to emerge. These recommendations or requirements are often expensive to implement and are not always based on risk assessment. It is important that they are based on evidence of associated improvement in control of infection or staff and patient safety. European disinfectant tests are also being introduced, but standardization and interpretation remain a problem, particularly in the development of more complex tests.

Finally, we would like also to express our thanks to Dr David Coates for his work on the previous edition (Ayliffe GAJ, Coates D and Hoffman PN. *Chemical Disinfection in Hospitals*, PHLS, 1993), much of which is included in the present edition. We are also grateful to the librarians at the HPA, patrticularly Potenza Atiogbe and David Keech for help with references, Dr John V Lee for advice on legionella control and Dr Paul Tearle for advice on safety.

PH
CB
GA

# 1 Principles of disinfection

The basic principle of infection control is to prevent pathogens reaching a susceptible site in sufficient numbers to cause an infection. Any process that reduces microbial numbers substantially on a route of infection transmission can contribute to the prevention of infection.

## Definitions

The terms used to describe the processes of reduction of microbial numbers are open to variable definitions. In this publication, we will use what we regard as consensus definitions as follows:

**Sterile** is the total absence of living organisms, in this context specifically of microbial life (or, in the case of viruses, of the ability to replicate).

**Sterilization** is a process used to render an object free from all living organisms with a high degree of quality assurance.

**Disinfection** is any process whereby the potential of an item to cause infection is removed by reducing the number of microorganisms present. Such a process may not necessarily eliminate all microorganisms, but can reduce them to a level such that they no longer are able to initiate infection. Numbers of bacterial spores may not necessarily be reduced. As the process of infection is the result of a combination of factors, any disinfection process must take into account the context in which it is being used. The term is applicable to the treatment of inanimate objects and materials and may also be applied to the treatment of the skin, mucous membranes and other body tissues and cavities. The main methods of achieving disinfection are by the use of heat or chemicals.

**Thermal disinfection** uses high temperatures to achieve disinfection.

A **disinfectant** is a chemical capable of achieving disinfection.

A **skin disinfectant** is a chemical disinfectant compatible with use on skin. The term **antiseptic** can also be used for skin disinfectants. Some skin disinfectants can also be used on mucous membranes or body tissues but consideration must be given to compatibility with the tissues to be treated.

The term **sterilant** is sometimes used for chemical disinfectants that reliably destroy bacterial spores as well as viruses and vegetative organisms. This form of sterilization does not have the same degree of sterility assurance as that achieved by physical methods (e.g. steam sterilization), recontamination can occur during post-process rinsing and items cannot be wrapped during liquid chemical sterilization.

**Cleaning** is a process which removes substantial amounts of any material that is not part of an item, including dust, soil, large numbers of microorganisms and the organic matter (e.g. faeces, blood) that protects them. Cleaning is usually a prerequisite to disinfection and sterilization. For chemical disinfection, it reduces both the bioburden and any organic matter that may shield the microbes or inactivate the disinfectant. For thermal disinfection and sterilization it both reduces bioburden and removes material that may coagulate and become firmly 'baked on' to an instrument. Some chemicals will also coagulate ('fix') proteins onto a surface.

The appreciation of the value of cleaning has been increased due to the prominence of the agents causing transmissible spongiform encephalopathies ('prions'). These agents cannot reliably be inactivated by conventional 'sterilization' processes and removal by cleaning plays a strategic role in routine infection control (though where there is a high risk of an instrument being contaminated, it should not be reused even if thoroughly cleaned).

**Decontamination** is a general term for the destruction or removal of microbial contamination to render an item safe. It can also cover removal of non-microbial matter. This will include methods of cleaning, disinfection and sterilization as appropriate.

## The processes

**Sterilization** is reliably achieved by physical methods such as heating in super-atmospheric steam in a steam sterilizer (autoclave), by dry heat in a hot air oven or by exposure to ionizing radiation. It can also be achieved by chemical methods such as ethylene oxide or gas plasma, as well as by combinations of thermal and chemical methods as found in low-temperature steam and formaldehyde. The most widely used sterilization method is steam sterilization. It is widely accepted that sterilization in centralized sterile service departments (SSDs) is the preferred route for sterilization in healthcare. These specialist departments have facilities and trained staff to carry out effective reprocessing of instruments. By use of specialist instrument washer-disinfectors, they can ensure that instruments are effectively cleaned and safe to handle; they can inspect instruments and organize repairs and servicing as necessary; they can wrap instruments correctly to enable maintenance of sterility on subsequent storage, sterilize the instrument packs in well-maintained porous load sterilizers (essential for wrapped items) and control the issue, traceability and maintenance of their stock. SSDs can also buy in and issue sterile, single-use instruments where this is appropriate.

## Thermal disinfection

Disinfection is most reliably achieved by moist heat. This will destroy all microorganisms except bacterial spores and the agents of transmissible spongiform encephalopathies ('prions'). Heat disinfection is one of the oldest processes in microbiology and, as pasteurization, goes back to Louis Pasteur. Thermal disinfection requires a specified temperature to be attained and held for a specified time. The higher the temperature, the shorter the time needed to achieve disinfection. Thermal disinfection can be combined with cleaning, as occurs in instrument or bedpan washer-disinfectors and laundering of fabrics. Thermal disinfection processes are widespread, not just in healthcare; the pasteurization of milk or the cooking of meat are both thermal disinfection processes of considerable public health significance.

In healthcare terms, thermal disinfection most commonly occurs in washer-disinfectors, variously for bedpans, instruments returned to SSDs, the reprocessing of anaesthetic equipment or laundry. Boiling water is still a common and effective means of achieving disinfection in regions of limited resources.

## Chemical disinfection

Chemical disinfection is inherently complicated because of the number and variety of factors that influence the antimicrobial activity of disinfectants: different microorganisms vary in their sensitivity to different disinfectants. Gram-positive bacterial species are usually sensitive, Gram-negative species less sensitive, mycobacteria relatively resistant and bacterial spores extremely resistant. Viruses also vary in their response to disinfectants, depending on their structure. Enveloped (lipid-containing) viruses are killed by most disinfectants but non-enveloped viruses tend to be more resistant.

Most disinfectants have a limited antimicrobial spectrum and very few are usefully sporicidal. Wherever possible, disinfectants should only be used on clean surfaces as they may fail to penetrate overlying soil such as blood or pus on instruments, and faecal residues on bedpans. Furthermore, they may be inactivated by organic matter, incompatible detergents, hard water and such materials as cork, rubber and plastic.

Many disinfectants are unstable and, after chemical breakdown has occurred, the solution may have little or no antimicrobial activity and may support the growth and proliferation of such versatile organisms as the pseudomonads. Hence it is essential that fresh dilutions of disinfectant are made up regularly in clean, preferably heat-treated, containers. Many disinfectants are also corrosive and irritant, and protective clothing and disposable gloves must be worn when handling them. In addition, items immersed in disinfectants usually require thorough rinsing before use and this can lead to recontamination.

The antimicrobial activity of disinfectants can be dependent upon pH; for example, glutaraldehyde is more active when alkaline. However, the active state of the compounds can also be the less stable form; for example, glutaraldehyde is more stable but less active at low pH. The compounds can be buffered to the most appropriate pH immediately before use, but will then have a limited use-life.

Different disinfectants vary markedly in the rate at which they kill microorganisms. Chlorine-based agents and alcohols act quickly, killing vegetative bacteria in as little as 1–2 minutes on clean surfaces, whereas some other disinfectants may take hours. Some disinfectants may just inhibit the growth of bacteria rather than kill them; i.e. they are bacteriostatic rather than bactericidal. Quaternary ammonium compounds, for example, are mainly bacteriostatic at very low concentrations, whereas at high concentrations they are bactericidal. From the above considerations it follows that chemical disinfection is often an uncertain procedure and that, wherever possible, physical disinfection methods are preferred.

There must be effective contact between the disinfectant and its target. The presence of organic matter can hamper penetration of the disinfectant and shield microbes from a chemical disinfectant. Air trapped in lumens in instruments will prevent contact between disinfectant and target. If items are put into disinfectant, they must be fully immersed and no air trapped within them.

## Cleaning

Efficient cleaning removes a high proportion of any microorganisms present, including bacterial spores, and in many hospital situations, thorough cleaning of the environment or items of equipment is adequate. For example, domestic cleaning and drying of hospital floors and walls is generally sufficient, and additional chemical disinfection is wasteful.

Similarly, in wards, cleaning of locker-tops, furniture, ledges and shelves is adequate, unless the surfaces are contaminated with potentially infectious material such as blood, faeces, pus or sputum. Some methods of cleaning, e.g. ultrasonic, are highly efficient; others, e.g. mop and bucket, are less so.

## Risk categories and levels of decontamination required

The choice of method of disinfection or sterilization depends on a number of factors, which include the type of material to be treated, the organisms involved, the time available for decontamination, and the risks to staff and patients. The infection risks to patients from equipment and the environment may be classified as shown in Table 1.

## Quality assurance and decontamination

### Thermal sterilization

The processes of thermal sterilization (i.e. by steam or by dry heat) are amenable to high levels of quality assurance, in essence by monitoring the time and temperature during a sterilization cycle. Such 'process control' is both more easy and more practical than an attempt to assure sterilization by sterility testing a proportion of items that have been through the process ('product control'). If the sterilizers are adequately maintained and sterilization cycle parameters are met, items can be released for use immediately ('parametric release'). If sterilization cycles are monitored only by use of biological indicators such as spore strips, items should not be released for use until the test spores have been given time to grow and have been shown to be non-viable.

Sterilization processes can often be used to provide excellent quality-assured decontamination for heat-tolerant items that may only require disinfection.

### Sterilization by ionizing irradiation

This is readily monitored. All that is needed is monitoring of the radiation dose; the time over which it is delivered is not relevant.

### Chemical sterilization

Processes such as ethylene oxide, low-temperature steam and formaldehyde, and gas plasma are multifactorial and less amenable to physical monitoring. For example, the process variables in sterilization by ethylene oxide primarily involve the concentration of ethylene oxide, the

**Table 1:** Risk categories and levels of decontamination required

| | Definition | Examples | Suitable methods |
|---|---|---|---|
| High risk | Items in close contact with a break in the skin or mucous membrane or introduced into a normally sterile body area | Surgical instruments, syringes and needles, intrauterine devices and associated equipment, dressings, urinary and other catheters | Sterilization is required. High-level disinfection, (i.e. disinfection which includes *M. tuberculosis* but not necessarily atypical mycobacteria or spores) may sometimes be acceptable if sterilization is not possible or practicable, e.g. arthroscopes and laparoscopes |
| Intermediate risk | Items in contact with intact mucous membranes | Respiratory equipment, gastroscopes, or other items contaminated with particularly virulent or readily transmissible organisms, or if the item is to be used on highly susceptible patients | Disinfection required |
| Low risk | Items in contact with normal and intact skin | Stethoscopes, washing bowls | Cleaning and drying usually adequate |
| Minimal risk | Items not in close contact with patients or their immediate surroundings | Floors, walls, ceilings and sinks | Cleaning and drying usually adequate |

temperature of the process, the time of exposure and the relative humidity. This combination of factors is best assessed by use of biological indicators (bacterial spores within a test piece which will require air removal and gas penetration). Loads should not be released until biological indicators are shown to be non-viable.

## Chemical disinfection

Chemical disinfection is less amenable to quality assurance monitoring than sterilization or thermal disinfection processes. The correct chemical must be used at the right concentration for an adequate exposure period in the absence of factors that may interfere with the process. With manual application, much depends on the diligence and training of the individual performing the process; even the same person may vary in diligence according to individual circumstances. With mechanical application in a chemical washer-disinfector, the method of application should not vary if the machine is properly maintained, but factors such as precleaning of an instrument and appropriate replacement of the disinfectant reservoir are problematic areas.

## Thermal disinfection

Thermal disinfection is easily monitored by checking the holding temperature achieved and the time that this is maintained. This tends to be checked periodically, rather than for every cycle as with steam sterilization.

## Further reading

Ayliffe GAJ, Fraise A, Mitchell K, Geddes A. (2000) *Control of Hospital Infection: A Practical Handbook*, 4th edn. Arnold, London. ISBN: 0340759119.

Block SS, ed. (2001) *Disinfection, Sterilization and Preservation*, 5th edn. Lippincott, Williams & Wilkins, Philadelphia. ISBN: 0683307401.

Fraise AP, Lambert P, Maillard J-Y, eds. (2003) *Russell, Hugo & Ayliffe's Principles and Practice of Disinfection, Preservation and Sterilization*, 4th edn. Blackwell Science, Oxford. ISBN: 1405101997.

Gardner JF, Peel MM. (1998) *Sterilization, Disinfection and Infection Control*, 3rd edn. Churchill Livingstone, Edinburgh. ISBN: 0443054355.

Microbiology Advisory Committee to the Department of Health. (1996) *Sterilization, Disinfection and Cleaning of Medical Equipment*. Department of Health, London. ISBN: 18858395186. [This document is updated periodically and current versions can be found on the website of the Medicines and Healthcare Products Regulatory Agency: http://www.mhra.gov.uk/].

# 2 Properties of chemical disinfectants

The general properties of important groups of disinfectants are given below. These properties may vary with individual products within a group and with the concentrations used. Some brands can include similar-sounding products with markedly different composition.

## Phenolics

**Uses:** Environment.

### Clear soluble phenolics
**Examples:** *Hycolin, Stericol* and *Clearsol.*

#### Properties
- Wide range of bactericidal activity, including mycobacteria.
- No practical sporicidal activity.
- Good fungicidal activity; limited virucidal activity, usually poor against non-enveloped viruses.
- Not readily inactivated by organic matter; absorbed by rubber and plastics.
- Contact with skin should be avoided.
- Taint food; do not use on food preparation surfaces or on equipment that may come into contact with skin or mucous membranes, particularly of infants.
- Contain detergents.
- Concentrates are stable but stability is reduced on dilution.
- Agents of choice for mycobacteria, including *Mycobacterium tuberculosis*, in the environment and laboratories.

### Black/white fluids
**Examples:** *Jeyes fluid, Lysol* and *Izal.*

### Properties
Properties of these fluids are generally similar to those of clear soluble phenolics listed above. Black/white fluids are cheaper than the latter, but have the disadvantage of being more harmful to skin, messy and strong smelling. They are rarely used within the healthcare setting.

## Chloroxylenol (para-chloro-meta-xylenol; 'PCMX')

### Properties
- Adequate activity against Gram-positive bacteria, but poor activity against some Gram-negative bacteria.
- Readily inactivated by a wide range of materials including organic matter and hard water.
- Non-corrosive and low irritancy.
- Not recommended for environment or instrument use in hospitals.

## Chlorine-based disinfectants

### Sodium hypochlorite
**Examples:** *Chloros, Domestos* and *Milton.*

### Properties
- Wide range of bactericidal including mycobacteria, virucidal and fungicidal activity.
- Sporicidal and mycobactericidal at concentrations at or over 1000 parts per million available chlorine (ppm av Cl).
- Disinfectant of choice for use against viruses, including blood-borne viruses.
- Rapid action.
- Inactivated by organic matter, particularly if used at low concentrations.
- Corrosive to some metals.
- Use-solutions should be freshly prepared.
- Care should be taken not to mix strong acids with hypochlorite because chlorine gas will be released.
- Hypochlorites should not be used in the presence of formaldehyde as one of the reaction products is carcinogenic.
- High concentrations are irritant and corrosive but low concentrations are of low toxicity.
- Useful for water treatment, in food preparation areas and milk kitchens, and as a laboratory disinfectant.
- Cheap.

Other hypochlorites, such as calcium hypochlorite, are used in some parts of the world. Properties are similar to sodium hypochlorite.

## Sodium dichloroisocyanurate (NaDCC)

Available as tablets, powders or granules.

**Examples:** *Presept, Sanichlor, Haz-Tab, Titan, Diversey detergent sanitizer.*

### Properties

- As for sodium hypochlorite but slightly less inactivation by organic matter and slightly less corrosive to metals.
- Often more convenient than hypochlorites.
- Undissolved tablets, powder and granules are very stable when stored dry, but unstable once in solution.

Accepted strengths for use of chlorine-based disinfectants are given in Table 2.

**Table 2:** Uses of chlorine-based disinfectants and recommended concentrations

| Use | Available chlorine | |
| --- | --- | --- |
| | % Hypochlorite* | Parts per million available chlorine (ppm av Cl) |
| Blood and body fluid spills | 1 | 10000 |
| Laboratory discard jars | 0.25 | 2500 |
| Environmental disinfection | 0.1 | 1000 |
| Disinfection of clean instruments | 0.05 | 500 |
| Infant feeding utensils, catering surfaces and equipment | 0.0125 | 125 |

* This is the concentration of the active component, *not* the dilution of the original product. Original products tend to vary between 10% and 0.1% hypochlorite (100 000 and 10 000 ppm av Cl).

## Chlorine dioxide

**Uses:** Heat-sensitive equipment, e.g. flexible endoscopes.

**Example:** *Tristel.*

### Properties

- Good bactericidal, virucidal, fungicidal and sporicidal activity.
- May be damaging to some materials.
- Unstable once prepared for use.
- Irritant to the skin and mucous membranes.

## Superoxidized water

**Uses:** Heat-sensitive equipment, e.g. flexible endoscopes.

**Example:** *Sterilox.*
This is a system that uses an electrolytic process to produce a disinfectant for use on the site of production. The solution can be piped over short distances, but should be used soon after production.

### Properties
- Rapid activity against bacteria, including mycobacteria, viruses, fungi and bacterial spores.
- Inactivated by organic matter.
- Solutions used once only and discarded.
- Unstable.
- May be damaging to some instrument components.
- Low toxicity and irritancy.

## Hydrogen peroxide and peroxygen compounds

### Peracetic acid
**Uses:** Heat-sensitive equipment, e.g. flexible endoscopes.

**Examples:** *Steris, Nu-Cidex, Perasafe, Perascope, Gigasept PA, Aperlan.*
Many different branded preparations are now available, but the activity of a particular concentration may vary depending on the preparation.

### Properties
- Good bactericidal, virucidal, fungicidal and sporicidal activity.
- May be damaging to some materials.
- Some formulations are unstable.
- Irritant to the skin and mucous membranes.
- Some products are unstable once prepared for use.

### Peroxide-based disinfectants
**Uses:** Equipment and environment.

**Examples:** Hydrogen peroxide and *Virkon.*

### Properties
- Wide range of bactericidal, virucidal and fungicidal activity.
- Inactivated by organic matter.
- Mycobactericidal and sporicidal activity variable.

- Corrosive to some metals.
- Often formulated with a detergent.
- Low toxicity and irritancy at use-dilutions.
- Sometimes used for disinfecting small spills and for laboratory equipment where other methods are impractical.
- Manufacturer's approval should be obtained before using on equipment where corrosion may present problems (e.g. laboratory equipment, centrifuges etc.).

## Diguanides (chlorhexidine)

**Uses:** Skin.

**Examples:** *Hibiscrub, Hibitane.*
Many different branded preparations are now available, but the activity of a particular concentration may vary depending on the preparation.

### Properties
- More active against Gram-positive than Gram-negative organisms.
- No activity against mycobacteria and bacterial spores.
- Good fungicidal activity.
- Limited activity against viruses.
- Low toxicity and irritancy at use-dilutions.
- Inactivated by organic matter, soap and anionic detergents.
- Most useful as disinfectants for skin and mucous membranes, but should not come into contact with brain, meninges, or middle ear.
- Mixtures of chlorhexidine and cetrimide are available prediluted and sterile in single-use sachets; commonly used for cleaning dirty wounds.

## Alcohol

**Uses:** Skin, environment and instruments.

**Examples:** Ethanol (including industrial methylated spirits) and isopropanol.

### Properties
- Good bactericidal (including mycobacteria) and fungicidal activity; not sporicidal.
- Ethanol is effective against enveloped viruses, but less effective against non-enveloped viruses.
- Isopropanol is effective against enveloped viruses but not against non-enveloped viruses.

- Rapid action.
- Volatile, useful as rapidly drying disinfectants for skin and surfaces.
- Must not be used undiluted (i.e. 100%). Usual concentrations are 70% for ethanol (90% for non-enveloped viruses) and 60–70% for isopropanol.
- Does not penetrate well into organic matter, especially protein-based, and should be used only on physically clean surfaces.
- Inflammable: care should be taken when using alcohols for environmental disinfection, on skin prior to diathermy or on electrical equipment.
- Can be used as a base for other bactericides (eg chlorhexidine, iodine, triclosan) for preoperative skin disinfection.
- Alcohol handrubs are a convenient alternative to handwashing.
- Alcohol wipes can be used for clean surface disinfection, though this allows limited exposure time. Immersion is preferable.

## Iodine and iodophors

**Uses:** Skin.

**Examples:** Aqueous iodine, tincture of iodine, *Betadine, Videne.*

### Properties
- Wide range of bactericidal, virucidal and fungicidal activity. Some activity against bacterial spores.
- Inactivated by organic matter.
- May corrode metals.
- Tincture of iodine and aqueous iodine solutions can cause skin reactions.
- Iodophors (e.g. *Betadine, Videne*) are complexes of iodine and carrier molecules: they do not stain skin and are non-irritant.

## Hexachlorophane (also known as hexachlorophene)

**Uses:** Skin.

**Example:** *Ster-Zac powder.*

### Properties
- More active against Gram-positive than Gram-negative bacteria.
- Little other microbicidal activity.
- Bacterial contamination of aqueous solutions can be a problem.
- Cutaneously absorbed hexachlorophane may be toxic to babies after repeated application of 3% hexachlorophane emulsions.

- Powders containing 0.33% hexachlorophane give some protection against colonization with *Staphylococcus aureus* in neonates, without significant toxicity risk.
- Good residual effect on skin.
- Can be used by adults for surgical hand disinfection or during staphylococcal outbreaks.

## Triclosan (also known as Irgasan)

**Uses:** Skin.

**Examples:** *Manusept, Aquasept, Ster-Zac bath concentrate* and *Cidal*.

### Properties
Triclosan disinfectants have properties and a spectrum of activity similar to the hexachlorophane disinfectants. Triclosan disinfectants exhibit no toxicity in neonates.

## Quaternary ammonium compounds (QACs) and ampholytic compounds

**Uses:** Environment and wounds.

**Examples:** *Roccal, Cetavlon* and *Tego*.

### Properties
- More active against Gram-positive than Gram-negative bacteria.
- No activity against bacterial spores.
- Variable mycobactericidal activity.
- Good fungicidal activity.
- Variable activity against viruses.
- Easily inactivated.
- Contamination and growth of Gram-negative bacilli in dilute solutions is possible.
- All have some detergent properties.
- Sterile QAC solutions with or without chlorhexidine may be used for cleaning dirty wounds.
- Some used in catering areas.
- Newer formulations may be suitable for environmental disinfection within healthcare.
- Ampholytic compounds (e.g. *Tego*) have properties similar to those of QACs.

# Aldehydes

## Glutaraldehyde

**Uses:** Heat-sensitive equipment, e.g. flexible endoscopes.

**Examples:** *Cidex, Asep* and *Totacide*.

### Properties

• Usually used as a 2% alkaline-buffered solution at room temperature.
• Wide range of bactericidal, virucidal and fungicidal activity.
• Slow activity against bacterial spores.
• Active against mycobacteria, but slower against M. *avium-intracellulare*.
• Irritant to eyes, skin and respiratory mucosa. Recognized as a respiratory irritant and asthmagen and causes contact dermatitis.
• Use must be limited to designated areas with appropriate exhaust-protective ventilation and personal protective equipment.
• Most preparations are non-damaging to metals and other materials.
• Little inactivation by organic matter, but penetrates slowly.
• A fixative; prior cleaning is always required.

## Formaldehyde

Formaldehyde is used mainly as a gaseous fumigant, particularly for laboratory safety cabinets. The humidity, temperature and formaldehyde concentration must be carefully controlled if fumigation is to be effective. Formaldehyde solution is too irritant to be used as a general disinfectant.

## Orthophthalaldehyde

**Uses:** Heat-sensitive equipment, e.g. flexible endoscopes.

**Example:** *Cidex OPA.*

### Properties

• Usually used at 0.55% at room temperature.
• Active against bacteria, including mycobacteria, viruses and fungi.
• No practical sporicidal activity.
• Little inactivation by organic material.
• Generates less vapour than glutaraldehyde, but general precautions for aldehydes as irritants and asthmagens are still appropriate.
• Irritant to the skin but not mucous membranes.
• Non-damaging to metals and other materials.

## Other aldehydes

Other aldehydes, e.g. succine dialdehyde (*Gigasept*), usually have properties similar to glutaraldehyde. With regard to safety, less is known about aldehydes other than formaldehyde and glutaraldehyde, but there are general concerns about the capacity of all aldehydes to be sensitizers and asthmagens.

## Further reading

Babb JR, Bradley CR. (2001) Choosing instrument disinfectants and processors. *British Journal of Infection* **2**, 10–13.

Block SS, ed. (2001) *Disinfection, Sterilization and Preservation*, 5th edn. Lippincott, Williams & Wilkins, Philadelphia. ISBN: 0683307401.

Fraise AP, Lambert P, Maillard J-Y, eds. (2003) *Russell, Hugo & Ayliffe's Principles and Practice of Disinfection, Preservation and Sterilization*, 4th edn. Blackwell Science, Oxford. ISBN: 1405101997.

Gardner JF, Peel MM. (1998) *Sterilization, Disinfection and Infection Control*, 3rd edn. Churchill Livingstone, Edinburgh. ISBN: 0443054355.

# 3 Disinfection policy

The purpose of a disinfection policy is to ensure that those responsible for disinfection are familiar with the disinfectants available, associated aspects of safety and procedures involved. The policy should be useful to all grades of staff and contractors working within the healthcare establishment and should improve cooperation between disciplines, e.g. nursing and domestic. It should define and standardize the methods (e.g. sterilization, disinfection and cleaning) for decontamination of equipment, of skin and of the inanimate environment. It should also ensure that the same disinfectants and concentrations are used for similar purposes throughout the establishment. The policy should reduce costs by eliminating unnecessary use of disinfectants and, by restricting the number of types available, should allow larger bulk purchases to be made at lower costs.

## Organization

The infection control committee is responsible for the formulation of the policy. Recommendations to the committee should be made on advice from the infection control officer/doctor, the infection control nurse, the microbiologist (if he/she is not the infection control officer), the pharmacist, the sterile services manager, the safety officer and the head biomedical scientist when the laboratory aspects are being discussed. Representatives of the users and the supplies officer should also be involved before the policy or changes are introduced.

Contractors, e.g. external cleaning companies, using disinfectants in healthcare establishments should obtain agreement on agents and their method of use from the infection control committee.

The infection control committee and sterile supplies department should be involved in the choice of new instruments and equipment in relation to methods of decontamination. Instruments should be heat-stable where possible. Manufacturers supplying instruments and equipment should provide prepurchase information on methods of decontamination. This is a requirement under the Medical Device Regulations (Statutory Instrument, 2002).

All requests for disinfectants should be approved by the pharmacist who will check that they are on the approved list. This applies particularly to restricted agents, such as glutaraldehyde. The pharmacist should also ascertain the compatibility of instruments and the processing equipment and to what extent personal protective clothing is required.

The use of disinfectants should be audited by occasional visits to wards and departments by the infection control team. This audit should include an assessment of the knowledge of staff as well as the use of disinfectants in practice. The policy should be reviewed annually and should be updated as necessary.

The policy may require temporary modification during outbreaks of infection and environmental disinfectants may be introduced (see Chapters 5 and 6). The outbreak committee should decide on the disinfectants to be used and methods of use on the advice of the infection control team and the pharmacist.

The infection control nurse should ensure that all relevant departments, particularly domestic, catering, laundry, sterile supplies, mortuary and laboratory, are aware of the policy and that suitable training is available for their staff. The importance of using correct dilutions, avoiding splashes to the skin and the wearing of appropriate types of glove when necessary should be stressed.

## Formulation

- List the purposes for which disinfectants are commonly used, e.g. environment, instruments, skin and mucous membrane.
- Eliminate the use of disinfectants where other methods are more appropriate, i.e.
  (a) where sterilization is essential, e.g. surgical instruments, implants, dressings and needles;
  (b) where heat can be used, e.g. washer-disinfectors for dirty surgical instruments, bowls, linen, crockery and cutlery, bedpans and urinals;
  (c) where cleaning alone is adequate, e.g. floors, walls and furniture;
  (d) where single-use items can be used economically, e.g. catheters, gloves and syringes.
- Select a disinfectant with an alternative for each remaining purpose.
- Arrange for the distribution of the disinfectant at the correct use-dilution whenever possible or in an easy-to-dilute presentation, such as NaDCC

tablets or sachets of liquid disinfectant. Most hospitals prefer to buy in disinfectants in the containers they will distribute them in. If they are diluted on site for distribution, the containers must be suitable and marked with any hazard warning necessary. If relevant, containers should be marked with a product expiry date.

## Choice of a disinfectant

• The disinfectant should have a wide spectrum of microbicidal activity and, if used for surface disinfection, should be rapid in action.
• It should not be readily neutralized by organic matter, soaps, hard water or plastics.
• It should be relatively non-corrosive at use-dilutions.
• It should be non-irritant if to be applied to the skin.
• It should be inexpensive.

A single disinfectant will not fulfil all these requirements, but usually a chlorine-based agent and a clear soluble phenolic or peroxygen will be sufficient for environmental disinfection. Narrow-spectrum disinfectants, such as quaternary ammonium compounds, should be avoided apart from occasions when a non-toxic agent may be required, e.g. in kitchens. Non-corrosive, wide-spectrum disinfectants may be needed for disinfection of medical instruments, particularly endoscopes; these were once generally disinfected with 2% glutaraldehyde but less toxic agents are now preferred (see Chapter 8). Seventy per cent alcohol may be required for rapid disinfection of some items, e.g. mercury-bulb thermometers. Compounds of low toxicity, e.g. chlorhexidine, povidone-iodine or 70% alcohol, will be required for skin disinfection.

A typical hospital disinfection policy is summarized in Appendix 1.

Policies covering areas within the community such as general and dental practices, health centres and nursing homes can be similar to those in hospitals. Other community applications such as schools, prisons and tattooing establishments will each require an individual approach to policy formulation taking into account the nature of infectious hazards, available resources and safety constraints. More detailed guidance may be found in the 'Further reading' sources given at the end of this chapter.

## Further reading

Ayliffe GAJ, Fraise AP, Geddes AM, Mitchell K, eds. (2000) *Control of Hospital Infection: A Practical Handbook*, 4th edn. Arnold, London. ISBN: 0340759119.

Coates D, Hutchinson DN. (1994) How to produce a hospital disinfectant policy. *Journal of Hospital Infection* **26**, 57–68.

Department of Health: Public Health Medicine Environmental Group. (1996) *Guidelines on the Control of Infection in Residential and Nursing Homes.* Department of Health, Wetherby.

Lawrence J, May D. (2002) *Infection Control in the Community.* Churchill Livingstone, Edinburgh. ISBN: 0443064067.

Pellowe CM, Pratt RJ, Harper P, Loveday HP, Robinson N, Jones SRLJ, MacRae ED. (2003) Prevention of healthcare-associated infections in primary and community care. *Journal of Hospital Infection* **55** (Suppl. 2), S5–S127.

Statutory Instrument 2002, Number 168. *The Medical Devices Regulations.* HMSO, London, 2002.

# 4 Thermal disinfection

## Properties

Heat disinfection will inactivate vegetative bacteria including mycobacteria, enveloped and non-enveloped viruses and fungi. It is poorly active against most bacterial spores. Wet heat transfers thermal energy better than dry heat. The temperatures used in heat disinfection are damaging to some materials and will act as a fixative for proteinaceous matter. Temperatures used are generally between 65°C and 100°C (boiling); the higher the temperature, the shorter the time needed to achieve disinfection. Hot water will injure body tissues; full-thickness skin burns result from transient contact at 80°C or over. The process is not significantly affected by the presence of organic matter. Heat disinfection can be used as a single process, as in an instrument boiler, or combined with another process, as in washer-disinfectors or fabric laundering.

Heat disinfection is one of the oldest processes in microbiology and, as either milk pasteurization or domestic cooking, the most widely used. In healthcare, it is a disinfection process of superior quality assurance compared to most chemical disinfection processes. As the efficacy of thermal disinfection depends on readily monitored parameters, principally temperature and time, each disinfection cycle can be assessed as it occurs. Such monitoring is usually carried out automatically during each disinfection cycle and a pass or fail indicated on completion. Items can be deemed disinfected if the cycle parameters are assessed as adequate, or failures can be noted and investigated. The accuracy of any self-assessment should be verified periodically by checking against calibrated external monitoring. Microbiological monitoring, by either the use of test organisms or sampling of disinfected items, is not normally done.

## Healthcare applications of heat disinfection

Thermal disinfection is widely used for hospital linen, bedpans and urine bottles, crockery and cutlery, suction bottles, surgical instruments and

**Table 3:** Thermal disinfection: UK times and temperatures

| Temperature | (°C) | Time |
|---|---|---|
| Washer-disinfectors | 65–70 | 10 min |
| | 73–78 | 3 min |
| | 80–85 | 1 min |
| | 90–95 | 12 s* |
| Laundry | 65 | 10 min |
| | 71 | 3 min |

*Whilst only 1 second is needed, the shortest time that this temperature can be measured in practice is 12 seconds.

respiratory equipment. The temperatures used range between 65 and 100°C. Generally the higher the temperature, the shorter the contact time. Automated thermal washer-disinfectors are available and these are preferred as they provide a standardized process and cleansing forms part of the cycle. A typical cycle consists of cleansing with detergent at <35°C, a main wash at 55°C, followed by thermal disinfection at a defined temperature and time, and drying.

The UK times and temperatures that are currently accepted to achieve thermal disinfection for various applications are given in Table 3.

## Instrument washer-disinfectors

These are usually located in departments that reprocess surgical instruments. Design parameters used in the UK are given in Health Technical Memorandum 2030 (NHS Estates Agency, 1997a). They are typically used to clean instruments and to make them safe to handle for inspection, maintenance and packing prior to steam sterilization. A typical automatic cycle comprises a cool (less than 35°C) initial wash to remove protein-based soils, a hot main wash (usually around 55°C), followed by rinses, during which the thermal disinfection occurs, followed by drying. Instrument washer-disinfectors can take the form of either a tunnel, in which instruments are transported and the washing and disinfecting occurs in sequential sections, or a single chamber.

Tunnel washer-disinfectors and chamber washer-disinfectors with two doors have the advantage that they can be loaded with instruments in a 'dirty' area and unloaded into a 'clean' area. Smaller cabinet machines are available which may be useful in post-mortem rooms and outlying clinics where a centralized service is not available.

## Washer-disinfectors for anaesthetic and respiratory equipment

These are similar to surgical instrument washer-disinfectors, but have internal connections that enable tubing to be flushed through. Design parameters used in the UK are given in Health Technical Memorandum 2030 (NHS Estates Agency, 1997a). As anaesthetic equipment does not need to be sterile, a washer-disinfector can be the sole decontamination process. Their use is declining with the increasing use of single-use anaesthetic equipment.

## Bedpan and urinal washer-disinfectors

These are also known as 'washer-disinfectors for human waste containers' and are intended to wash and disinfect the containers as well as to dispose of their contents. Design parameters used in the UK are given in Health Technical Memorandum 2030 (NHS Estates Agency, 1997a). Separate emptying of the containers before loading them into the washer-disinfector should not need to occur. After loading, the washer-disinfector should have an automatic cycle comprising an initial wash at less than 35°C, then a wash which may or may not include detergent and a descaling agent, followed by rinses, the last of which should contain the heat disinfection phase. Some machines can have a subsequent cooling phase or drying phase, but these are not common. With most cycles, natural drying is aided by the heat gained during the final hot rinse. Bedpan and urinal washer-disinfectors should be located in a ward's dirty utility room ('sluice').

### Controls

The verification and testing of instrument, anaesthetic equipment and bedpan washer-disinfectors is detailed in Health Technical Memorandum 2030 (NHS Estates Agency, 1997b) and BS 2745 (British Standards Institution, 1993). Verification comprises a schedule of periodic monitoring of cycle parameters designed not only to check that the cycles proceed as intended, but also to verify that the machine's self-monitoring of parameters is accurate. The cleaning capabilities of a washer-disinfector can be tested by observation of removal of an artificial soil applied to items in the load and also by detection of residual natural soils such as the detection of protein left on instruments by the use of ninhydrin (which will be turned purple by traces of protein).

Washers used in laboratories and post-mortem rooms may not require the same level of testing as those used for surgical instruments.

## Healthcare laundry

Heat disinfection is the preferred method for the decontamination of healthcare linens between uses. The temperatures used and the holding times at those temperatures are given in Table 3 (NHS Executive, 1995). These process parameters should be the same for all heat-tolerant linen, irrespective of whether it is classed as used, soiled or infectious (see Chapter 6 for details).

## Instrument boilers

These are self-heating vessels in which instruments can be immersed in boiling water. Instruments must be cleaned as a separate procedure before immersion in the boiler. If this does not occur, proteinaceous matter will be heat-coagulated and fixed onto instruments. Instrument boilers do not have thermostats or timers, so water temperature has to be judged visually (by observation of boiling) and timing has to be done separately by the operator. Immersion in boiling water for 5 minutes will kill all microorganisms except bacterial spores and provides a generous safety margin. Washer-disinfectors have superior quality assurance and should be used where resources will permit. However instrument boilers give superior disinfection to the use of chemical disinfection, so their use is appropriate in areas of severely limited resources, such as primary care in developing countries.

## References

British Standards Institution. (1993) BS 2745-1:1993 *Washer-disinfectors for medical purposes. Specification for general requirements.* British Standards Institution, London.

NHS Estates Agency. (1997a) *Washer-disinfectors: Design considerations. Health technical memorandum 2030.* NHS Estates, Leeds. ISBN: 0113220693.

NHS Estates Agency. (1997b) *Washer-disinfectors: Validation and verification. Health technical memorandum 2030.* NHS Estates, Leeds. ISBN: 0113220715.

NHS Executive. (1995) *Health Service Guidelines: Hospital laundry arrangements for used and infected linen.* HSG(95)18. Department of Health, London.

## Further reading

British Standards Institution. (1993) BS 2745-2:1993 *Washer-disinfectors for medical purposes. Specification for human waste container washer-disinfectors.* British Standards Institution, London.

British Standards Institution. (1993) BS 2745-3:1993 *Washer-disinfectors for medical purposes. Specification for washer-disinfectors except those used for processing human-waste containers and laundry.* British Standards Institution, London.

Fraise AP, Lambert P, Maillard J-Y, eds. (2003) *Russell, Hugo & Ayliffe's Principles and Practice of Disinfection, Preservation and Sterilization,* 4th edn. Blackwell Science, Oxford. ISBN: 1405101997.

NHS Estates Agency. (1997) *Washer-disinfectors: Operational management. Health technical memorandum 2030.* NHS Estates, Leeds. ISBN: 0113220707.

# 5 Organisms of special significance

Bacteria and viruses vary in their resistance to chemical and thermal disinfection (Table 4). Vegetative bacteria (i.e. bacteria in their normal replicating state) are generally sensitive to inactivation by most disinfectants. Gram-positive bacteria are sensitive to most disinfectants. Some of the environmental Gram-negative bacteria (such as pseudomonads and achromobacter) can be less sensitive to some disinfectants whereas others (such as the Enterobacteriaceae) are sensitive to most disinfectants.

Some bacteria can form spores, highly stable forms with thick walls that can survive in the environment for years, and are resistant to many commonly used environmental disinfectants and moderate degrees of moist heat such as 80°C; some can survive boiling water for hours. (Spore-forming bacteria in their normal vegetative state are as sensitive to inactivation as other vegetative bacteria. Statements such as 'kills spore-forming bacteria' do not necessarily refer to inactivation of bacterial spores.) Mycobacteria show moderate resistance to disinfectants but are sensitive to heat. Fungi and fungal spores are sensitive to inactivation by most disinfectants. Some viruses have lipid-based envelopes that are essential to their infectivity. As these envelopes are easily disrupted by chemical disinfectants, enveloped viruses are sensitive to inactivation by most disinfectants. Viruses without these envelopes are resistant to some disinfectants.

There is no correlation between pathogenicity and resistance to chemical or thermal inactivation. There is no evidence to show that bacteria with multiple antibiotic resistances are significantly less sensitive to environmental chemical disinfectants. Where concerns exist about decreased sensitivity of some Gram-positive bacteria, these are discussed under the relevant specific heading. Details of the microbicidal ranges of individual disinfectants are given in Chapter 2.

**Table 4:** Microbial resistance to inactivation

| Generalized microbial resistance to chemical disinfectants | |
|---|---|
| Extreme resistance | Prions |
| High resistance | Bacterial spores |
| Moderately resistant | Mycobacteria |
| | Non-enveloped viruses |
| Moderately sensitive | Fungal spores |
| | Gram-negative bacilli |
| Sensitive | Gram-positive cocci |
| | Enveloped viruses |
| | Fungi |

| Generalized microbial resistance to thermal disinfection | |
|---|---|
| Extreme resistance | Prions |
| High resistance | Bacterial spores |
| Moderately sensitive | Enterococci |
| Sensitive | Mycobacteria |
| | Gram-negative bacilli |
| | Gram-positive cocci |
| | Enveloped viruses |
| | Non-enveloped viruses |
| | Fungi and fungal spores |

# Bacterial spores

Spores are formed from vegetative forms by the bacterial genera *Clostridium* (anaerobes) and *Bacillus* (aerobes). Both the spores and vegetative forms are commonly found in soil and in the gastrointestinal tracts of humans and other mammals. Bacterial spores are resistant to many disinfectants in common use and many can survive boiling for prolonged periods. Incineration, autoclaving and dry heat at high temperatures are the most reliable methods of killing spores. Ethylene oxide and gas plasma systems are also sporicidal. Some chemical disinfectants, principally chlorine-based disinfectants, peracetic acid, glutaraldehyde and superoxidized water, are capable of inactivating bacterial spores, but the quality assurance of this process is lower than that of heat sterilization processes. Chemical sporicides should only be used where heat sterilization is not feasible.

*Clostridium difficile* is currently a particular problem in healthcare as the cause of an antibiotic-associated colitis, with symptoms ranging from diarrhoea to a more severe pseudomembranous colitis. Heavy contamination of the environment can occur, particularly from incontinent patients with antibiotic-associated diarrhoea. The organism forms spores which survive well in the environment. It can be killed by steam sterilization and sporicidal chemical disinfectants. It is more sensitive than other clostridia to 2% glutaraldehyde which is sporicidal in 5–20 minutes (Dyas & Das, 1985; Rutala et al., 1993). Removal of its spores from the environment can be difficult and repeated thorough cleaning is recommended. Efficient cleaning of bedpans is particularly significant since heating to 70–80°C in bedpan washer-disinfectors will not kill the spores. Following removal of excess organic matter, the environment can be disinfected with a chlorine-based disinfectant (1000 ppm av Cl) during outbreak situations or for terminal disinfection (Wilcox et al., 2003; Mayfield et al., 2000), but this is corrosive and may cause damage. The organism is mainly transferred on the hands, and the wearing of gloves and thorough washing of hands with soap and water is important. The commonly used skin disinfectants, including alcohol, are ineffective.

The spores of *Bacillus subtilis* are more resistant to disinfectants than most bacterial spores and are commonly used for testing the sporicidal activity of disinfectants. Two per cent alkaline glutaraldehyde can kill one million *B. subtilis* spores in 2–3 hours (Babb et al., 1980), although 10 hours is sometimes recommended based on the official test used in the USA. Orthophthalaldehyde (OPA) is less effective against spores. Sodium hypochlorite solutions, buffered to pH 7.6, are rapidly sporicidal (Death & Coates, 1979), but may corrode instruments. Other agents, such as peracetic acid, chlorine dioxide and superoxidized water are effective against one million *B. subtilis* spores in 5–10 minutes (Selkon et al., 1999; Shetty et al., 1999; Coates, 2001) and are less corrosive than other chlorine-based disinfectants.

*Bacillus anthracis* spores are of current interest as they could be used in bioterrorism or warfare. They survive well in the environment and in general show similar resistance to chemical disinfection as other *Bacillus* species. Severe infections are mainly acquired from inhaled aerosols. Steam sterilization is the method of choice for decontaminating equipment. Contaminated surfaces should be disinfected with a chlorine-based disinfectant at 1000 ppm av Cl.

## Mycobacteria

Tuberculosis is still a major disease throughout the world and the number of strains of tubercle bacilli (*Mycobacterium tuberculosis*) resistant to commonly used chemotherapeutic agents continues to increase. There has also been an increase in infections caused by other mycobacteria ('atypical mycobacteria'), most of which are of environmental origin. *Mycobacterium avium-intracellulare* infection occurs in immunosuppressed patients, particularly in those infected with human immunodeficiency virus (HIV). *M. chelonae* and *M. fortuitum* have been responsible for occasional clinical infections or pseudoepidemics when specimens are generated using contaminated bronchoscopes.

*Mycobacterium tuberculosis* is mainly transmitted by the airborne route but because of its resistance to drying, surfaces could be potential vehicles of transmission. It is more resistant to chemical disinfectants than other non-sporing bacteria, but less so than spores. It is equally susceptible to thermal disinfection as non-sporing bacteria. Items contaminated with discharges from tuberculous patients should be disposed of by incineration or by autoclaving whenever possible. Exposure to wet heat with an appropriate time/temperature relationship (see Chapter 4), <2% alkaline glutaraldehyde, 1–2% clear soluble phenolic for 20 minutes, 0.55% OPA, peracetic acid, chlorine dioxide and superoxidized water for 5–10 minutes (Rutala *et al.*, 1991; Holton *et al.*, 1994; Griffiths *et al.*, 1999; Selkon *et al.*, 1999) should all kill tubercle bacilli on clean equipment such as endoscopes (see Chapter 8, Table 6). Chlorine-based disinfectants at 1000–10 000 ppm av Cl or a clear soluble phenolic at a concentration for dirty conditions may be used for disinfecting surfaces in the post-mortem room, laboratory or elsewhere.

Some mycobacteria such as *M. avium-intracellulare* are more resistant to glutaraldehyde (Collins, 1986; Griffiths *et al.*, 1999) and exposure for at least 1 hour is recommended if an atypical mycobacterial infection is suspected, or is likely, for example in AIDS patients. The other agents and heat mentioned above should be effective in the times quoted for tubercle bacilli. Multiple drug-resistant *Mycobacterium tuberculosis* is no more resistant to thermal or chemical disinfection than drug-sensitive strains.

*Mycobacterium chelonae* resistant to 2% glutaraldehyde has been isolated from washer-disinfectors that used glutaraldehyde as the disinfectant. The strain is sensitive to the other recommended agents (van Klingeren & Pullen, 1993; Griffiths *et al.*, 1997). For this reason, an agent other than that routinely used for endoscope decontamination is recommended for routine disinfection of endoscope washer-disinfectors.

## Staphylococcus aureus

*Staphylococcus aureus* is the commonest cause of infection in clean surgical wounds. Resistance to benzyl penicillin was described soon after it was introduced into clinical practice in the 1940s and resistance has emerged in some strains to most subsequently introduced antibiotics. Methicillin-resistant *Staph. aureus* (MRSA), also resistant to other penicillinase-resistant penicillins and cephalosorins, was reported in the 1960s and such multiresistant MRSAs have become a problem in many countries since then. Some strains of epidemic MRSA have been reported as being less sensitive to some skin disinfectants (e.g. quaternary ammonium disinfectants, triclosan and chlorhexidine) than antibiotic-sensitive strains (Brumfitt *et al.*, 1985; Suller & Russell, 1999). In other studies, no difference was shown between MRSA and methicillin-sensitive *Staph. aureus* (Bamber & Neal, 1999).

Such decreased sensitivities are sometimes termed 'resistance', but they are mainly low level (i.e. a decreased sensitivity rather than true resistance) and are unlikely to be of clinical significance. The agents can still be recommended for treating MRSA carriers and for hand disinfection following contact with these patients (Cookson *et al.*, 1991). However, occasionally a change to an alternative agent may be worth consideration following apparent failures with one agent, e.g. the use of triclosan instead of chlorhexidine or povidone-iodine for bathing MRSA carriers.

MRSA survives well in the environment, as do other *Staph. aureus*, but the routine use of disinfectants during outbreaks remains controversial since recontamination of the environment is likely to occur if a room remains occupied by infected patients or carriers. Routine cleaning with detergent during a room's occupation is usually considered adequate. However, increased cleaning, especially removal of dust with a vacuum cleaner, has been associated with a reduction in MRSA (Rampling *et al.*, 2001). Terminal disinfection after the discharge of an MRSA patient is rational, although there is little evidence that this reduces the risk of infection to the next occupant more than thorough cleaning would. There is no evidence that antibiotic-resistant *Staph. aureus* acquires resistance to environmental disinfectants used in hospitals, and phenolics, chlorine-based agents and peroxygen compounds can be used in the recommended concentrations, if indicated. Staphylococci are also killed at thermal disinfection temperatures used in washer-disinfectors (see Chapter 4, Table 3).

## Coagulase-negative staphylococci

These have become of increasing importance in recent years, causing infections in prostheses and intravascular catheters. They have often acquired resistance to the same antibiotics as *Staph. aureus*, but spread less readily from patient to patient than epidemic MRSA and outbreaks are rare. Although studies are limited, coagulase-negative staphylococci appear to be sensitive to the same chemical and thermal disinfection processes as MRSA. Routine environmental cleaning without disinfection should be adequate.

## Vancomycin-resistant enterococci (VRE)

Enterococci are part of the normal flora of the intestinal tract and are commonly of low virulence. They are causes of urinary and biliary tract infection and pelvic sepsis, usually in association with other organisms. Invasive infections and outbreaks occur mainly in intensive care and units containing immunosuppressed patients. In recent years resistance has emerged to commonly used antibiotics, including quinolones and high levels of aminoglycosides, and plasmids controlling beta-lactamases have increased their resistance to penicillins and cephalosporins. The emergence of multiresistant strains, mainly *Enterococcus faecium*, to glycopeptides (vancomycin and teicoplanin) was reported in 1988, increasing the problem of treating severe infections and controlling outbreaks.

Enterococci survive well in the inanimate environment and spread mostly on the hands of staff, but also on equipment such as bedpans, toilets, fluidized microsphere beds, electronic thermometers and possibly colonoscopes and sigmoidoscopes. There is little evidence that routine disinfection of the environment is necessary to control spread, but thorough daily cleaning is necessary. As with MRSA, terminal disinfection should be considered in outbreaks of highly resistant strains.

Enterococci are readily killed by most disinfectants, such as phenolics, chlorine-based compounds and 70% alcohol in less than 5 minutes and there is no obvious correlation between antibiotic resistance and resistance to biocides. The usual hand disinfection agents are mainly effective, although aqueous chlorhexidine has been reported as less effective against vancomycin-resistant strains than vancomycin-sensitive strains (Kampf *et al.*, 1999), but not in all studies (Anderson *et al.*, 1997; Suller & Russell, 1999; Sakagami *et al.*, 2002). Disinfection of the hands with an alcoholic solution is commonly recommended.

Enterococci are less sensitive to heat disinfection than most other vegetative bacteria. Most enterococcal strains are killed by temperatures in excess of 70°C but some strains require 80°C for 3 minutes (Bradley & Fraise, 1996). A combination of effective removal by cleaning and killing by heat can usually be obtained in effective washer-disinfectors with standard thermal disinfection cycles (see Chapter 4, Table 3).

# Legionella

*Legionella pneumophila* and other strains of legionella are Gram-negative bacilli that can normally be found in soil and surface water and are sometimes present in building water supplies, including those of hospitals and hotels. They can be transmitted from shower heads, spa pools, medical equipment such as humidifiers and nebulizers, and hot or cold water supplies in hospitals. (Cleaning and maintenance of spa pools presents such difficulties that their use in hospitals is not recommended.) Immunocompromised patients are particularly vulnerable. Major community outbreaks are usually associated with wet cooling towers serving air conditioning systems in large buildings; major outbreaks in hospitals are usually associated with hot water systems. Infections are transmitted by aerosols and do not spread from person to person. Prevention is important and particular care is required in high-risk units. Good design and maintenance of wet cooling towers, water distribution systems and relevant items of medical equipment is required. However, legionellae may be protected from biocides by biofilms or they may survive within environmental amoebae.

Cleaning and disinfection of cooling towers should be carried out at least twice yearly (Health and Safety Commission, 2002) and treatment with appropriate biocides should reduce legionellae to small numbers. Water tanks should be inspected for sludge (cold tanks) and scale (hot tanks) annually, and cleaned or descaled where necessary (Health and Safety Commission, 2002). Hot water tanks should preferably be kept at 60°C and cold water at 20°C or less. 'Dead legs' in water distribution systems should be eliminated and hot and cold pipes should be kept separate and lagged to avoid transfer of heat between them. The elimination of legionella from water systems depends mainly on removal of biofilm and debris, and either chlorination or raising the water temperature. Chlorination of a cooling tower may be achieved by raising the chlorine level to 5 mg per litre (ppm av Cl) for several hours. Higher levels of 50 mg per litre in cold water tanks are sometimes recommended, but corrosion is likely to occur with high chlorine levels. Other treatments such as chlorine dioxide and copper–silver ionization are also now being used to control legionellae (Health and Safety Commission, 2002). Heating the hot water system to give outlet water temperatures of at least 52°C is another possibility, but scalding can occur, particularly in the elderly, so the use of thermostatic mixers at outlets is recommended if this option is adopted. Building maintenance to control legionella is extensively covered elsewhere (Health and Safety Commission, 2002; The Chartered Institution of Building Services Engineers, 2002). Medical equipment

should be decontaminated with hypochlorites or by heat, although sometimes single-use items will be preferred.

## Viruses

Although viruses vary in their resistance to disinfectants, they will be
inactivated by the usual methods of sterilization and by water at temperatures of 70°C or above. Enveloped viruses are sensitive to disinfectants in routine use but non-enveloped viruses show greater resistance
(Sattar *et al.*, 1989; Tyler *et al.*, 1990) (see Chapter 2 for details of individual disinfectants). Phenolics, quaternary ammonium compounds and
chlorhexidine show varying activity and are usually not recommended
for routine disinfection in hospitals if an antiviral effect is required. Aldehydes, chlorine based compounds (including chlorine dioxide) and peracetic acid in appropriate concentrations are effective against all viruses.
Iodine and peroxygen compounds are less corrosive alternatives that may
be used on clean surfaces. Superoxidized water is also effective against
viruses and may be useful for decontaminating clean instruments, but is
readily inactivated by organic matter. Non-enveloped viruses are resistant
to isopropanol and moderately resistant to 70% ethanol; 85–90% ethanol
is more effective, but physical removal by handwashing is preferable. HIV
is an enveloped virus and is sensitive to most disinfectants in routine use
(Sattar *et al.*, 1994). Hepatitis viruses (B and C) are thought to be inactivated
by alkaline 2% glutaraldehyde, chlorine-based agents, peracetic acid and
70% ethanol in 5–10 minutes (Deva *et al.*, 1996). Hepatitis A spreads by
the faecal–oral route and is thought to be one of the most resistant viruses
to disinfectants, but is sensitive to aldehydes, chlorine-based compounds
and peracetic acid (Mbithi *et al.*, 1990).

The viruses of Lassa, Ebola and Marburg and other haemorrhagic
fevers, smallpox and rabies viruses are inactivated by most disinfectants.
Chlorine-based agents are commonly recommended for routine use. Terminal disinfection of rooms, wards, ambulances and blood spillage is
described by the Advisory Committee on Dangerous Pathogens (1996).

There have been no data published at the time of writing on the disinfectant susceptibilities of the coronavirus causing severe acute respiratory
syndrome (SARS). However, the virus is enveloped and should be susceptible to most disinfectants. A chlorine-based disinfectant is the agent
of choice.

Washer-disinfectors and laundry washing machines at temperatures
described in Chapter 4 should remove or inactivate viruses. Although
the precise temperatures required for inactivating hepatitis viruses are

unknown, thorough washing in a machine at 70–80°C should reduce risks of transmission.

## Prions

Prions are abnormal protease-resistant protein particles which accumulate in the central nervous system in Creutzfeldt–Jakob disease (CJD), Kuru, bovine spongiform encephalopathy (BSE), scrapie in sheep and other transmissible spongiform encephalopathies in humans and animals. Infection has been transmitted from contaminated growth hormone preparations, corneal implants and rarely from surgical instruments used on patients with CJD. BSE is thought to be transferred to humans from eating material from infected cattle, and the new disease in humans, variant Creutzfeldt–Jacob disease (vCJD), was first identified in 1996. In addition to the central nervous system, prions have been identified in the lymphoreticular system, including the tonsils of patients with vCJD, but not sporadic CJD. There is no evidence as yet of transfer of vCJD to patients or staff in hospitals.

### Decontamination of instruments

Prions are very resistant to inactivation by heat and chemicals. Tests for effectiveness of disinfectants usually involve brain tissue which may provide protection to the prions and increase the difficulties of interpretation of results. However, prions appear to be resistant to aldehydes, alcohols, phenolics, peracetic acid, peroxides, iodophors, quaternary ammonium compounds, ethylene oxide, UV light, ionizing radiation and both dry and moist heat at the usual sterilizing temperatures and times. Accepted decontamination processes include 20 000 ppm av Cl from sodium hypochlorite (but not from NaDCC) for 1 hour, 2M sodium hydroxide for 1 hour, autoclaving at 134–137°C for 18 minutes, or six sequential cycles of 134–137°C for 3 minutes each (Taylor, 2003). Decontamination with sodium hydroxide and heat are known to be only partially effective. Histological samples can be exposed to 96% formic acid for 1 hour after routine fixation.

Various body tissues are thought to have different risks of infectivity of CJD and vCJD:

- tissue from the brain, spinal cord and posterior eye is thought to have high infectivity;
- tissue from the anterior eye and olfactory epithelium in CJD and the anterior eye and olfactory epithelium and lymphoid tissue in vCJD is thought to have medium infectivity;
- other tissues are thought to have low infectivity.

The following actions are recommended according to the likelihood of a patient having CJD or vCJD and the infectivity of the tissues involved in surgery. Patients can be classified as having definite, probable or possible CJD and vCJD. Iatrogenic and genetic risk factors should also be established (Advisory Committee on Dangerous Pathogens; Spongiform Encephalopathy Advisory Committee, 2003).

- Where the likelihood of prions being present is definite or probable and tissue involved in surgery is high or medium infectivity, single-use instruments should be used wherever possible; all non-single-use surgical instruments used should be destroyed. Where the tissues involved are not high or medium risk, instruments need no special precautions for reprocessing.
- Where the patient has a 'possible' status for CJD or vCJD, instruments in contact with high- and medium-infectivity tissues should be quarantined until a definite diagnosis is available, and then destroyed or reprocessed as appropriate. Where the tissues involved are not high or medium risk, instruments need no special precautions for reprocessing.
- Where the patient is at iatrogenic or genetic risk of CJD or vCJD, and tissues involved have high or medium infectivity, non-single-use surgical instruments used should be destroyed. Where the tissues involved are not high or medium risk, instruments need no special precautions for reprocessing.

Endoscopes cannot be decontaminated effectively. A number of endoscopes are kept at centres in the UK specifically for use on patients with confirmed CJD.

Further guidance on infection control in the context of CJD and prions is published by the Department of Health (Advisory Committee on Dangerous Pathogens; Spongiform Encephalopathy Advisory Committee, 2003).

The use of all non-single-use invasive surgical instruments and endoscopes should be capable of being traced (Department of Health, 1999). If instruments are used on patients who are later diagnosed as being suspect or probable CJD or vCJD cases, this makes it possible to identify and quarantine or destroy these instruments, and to identify any patients subsequently exposed via instruments.

## References

Advisory Committee on Dangerous Pathogens. (1996) *Management and Control of Viral Haemorrhagic Fevers.* The Stationery Office, London. ISBN: 0113218605.

Advisory Committee on Dangerous Pathogens; Spongiform Encephalopathy Advisory Committee. (2003) *Transmissible spongiform encephalopathy agents: safe working and the prevention of infection.* [Currently only available from the Department of Health website at: http://www.dh.gov.uk].

Anderson RL, Carr JH, Bond WW, Favero MS. (1997) Susceptibility of vancomycin-resistant enterococci to environmental disinfectants. *Infection Control and Hospital Epidemiology* **18**, 195–199.

Babb JR, Bradley CR, Ayliffe GAJ. (1980) Sporicidal activity of glutaraldehyde and hypochlorites and other factors influencing their selection for the treatment of medical equipment. *Journal of Hospital Infection* **1**, 63–75.

Bamber AI, Neal TJ. (1999) An assessment of triclosan susceptibility in methicillin-resistant and methicillin-sensitive *Staphylococcus aureus. Journal of Hospital Infection* **41**, 107–109.

Bradley CR, Fraise AP. (1996) Heat and chemical resistance of enterococci. *Journal of Hospital Infection* **34**, 191–196.

Brumfitt W, Dixson S, Hammilton-Miller JMT. (1985) Resistance to antiseptics in methicillin and gentamicin resistant *Staphylococcus aureus. Lancet* **1**, 1442–1443.

The Chartered Institution of Building Services Engineers. (2002) *TM 13: Minimising the risk of Legionnaires' disease.* The Chartered Institution of Building Services Engineers, London. ISBN: 1903287235.

Coates D. (2001) An evaluation of the use of chlorine dioxide (Tristel One-Shot) in an automated washer/disinfector (Medivator) fitted with a chlorine dioxide generator for decontamination of flexible endoscopes. *Journal of Hospital Infection* **48**, 55–65.

Collins FM. (1986) Bactericidal activity of alkaline glutaraldehyde solutions against a number of atypical mycobacterial species. *Journal of Applied Bacteriology* **61**, 247–251.

Cookson BD, Bolton MC, Platt JH. (1991) Chlorhexidine resistance in methicillin-resistant *Staphylococcus aureus* or just an elevated MIC? An in vitro and in vivo assessment. *Antimicrobial Agents and Chemotherapy* **35**, 1997–2002.

Death JE, Coates D. (1979) Effect of pH on sporicidal and microbicidal activity of buffered mixtures of alcohol and sodium hypochlorite. *Journal of Clinical Pathology* **32**, 148–153.

Department of Health. (1999) *Variant Creutzfeldt–Jakob disease—minimising the risk of transmission.* Health Service Circular HSC1999/178. Department of Health, London.

Deva AK, Vickery K, Zou L, West RH, Harris JP, Cossart YE. (1996) Establishment of an in-use method for evaluating disinfection of surgical instruments using the duck hepatitis B model. *Journal of Hospital Infection* **33**, 119–130.

Dyas A, Das BC. (1985) The activity of glutaraldehyde against *Clostridium difficile*. *Journal of Hospital Infection* **6**, 41–45.

Griffiths PA, Babb JR, Bradley CR, Fraise AP. (1997) Glutaraldehyde-resistant *Mycobacterium chelonae* from endoscope washer disinfectors. *Journal of Applied Microbiology* **82**, 519–526.

Griffiths PA, Babb JR, Fraise AP. (1999) Mycobactericidal activity of selected disinfectants using a quantitative suspension test. *Journal of Hospital Infection* **41**, 111–121.

Health and Safety Commission (2002) *L8. Legionnaires' disease: the control of legionella bacteria in water systems: approved code of practice and guidance*. Health and Safety Commission, London. ISBN: 0717617726.

Holton J, Nye P, McDonald V. (1994) Efficacy of selected disinfectants against mycobacteria and cryptosporidium. *Journal of Hospital Infection* **27**, 105–115.

Kampf G, Hoper M, Went C. (1999) Efficacy of hand disinfectants against vancomycin-resistant enterococci in vitro. *Journal of Hospital Infection* **42**, 143–150.

van Klingeren B, Pullen W. (1993) Glutaraldehyde-resistant mycobacteria from endoscope washers. *Journal of Hospital Infection* **25**, 147–149.

Mayfield JL, Leet T, Miller J, Mundy LM. (2000) Environmental control to reduce transmission of *Clostridium difficile*. *Clinical Infectious Diseases* **31**, 995–1000.

Mbithi JN, Springthorpe VS, Sattar SA. (1990) Chemical disinfection of hepatitis A virus on environmental surfaces. *Applied and Environmental Microbiology* **56**, 3601–3604.

Rampling A, Wiseman S, Davis L, Hyett AP, Payne GC, Cornaby AJ. (2001) Evidence that hospital hygiene is important in the control of methicillin-resistant *Staphylococcus aureus*. *Journal of Hospital Infection* **49**, 109–116.

Rutala WA, Cole EC, Wannamaker MS, Weber DJ. (1991) Inactivation of *Mycobacterium tuberculosis* and *Mycobacterium bovis* by 14 hospital disinfectants. *American Journal of Medicine* **91** (Suppl. B), 267S–271S.

Rutala WA, Gergen MF, Weber DJ. (1993) Inactivation of clostridium spores by disinfectants. *Infection Control and Hospital Epidemiology* **14**, 36–39.

Sakagami Y, Kajimura K. (2002) Bactericidal activities of disinfectants against vancomycin-resistant enterococci. *Journal of Hospital Infection* **50**, 140–144.

Sattar SA, Springthorpe VS, Karim Y, Loro P. (1989) Chemical disinfection of non-porous inanimate surfaces experimentally contaminated with four human pathogenic viruses. *Epidemiology and Infection* **102**, 493–505.

Sattar SA, Springthorpe VS, Conway B, Xu Y. (1994) Inactivation of the human immunodeficiency virus: an update. *Reviews in Medical Microbiology* **5**, 139–150.

Selkon JB, Babb JR, Morris R. (1999) Evaluation of the antimicrobial activity of a new superoxidized water, 'Sterilox', for the disinfection of endoscopes. *Journal of Hospital Infection* **41**, 59–70.

Shetty N, Srinivasan S, Holton J, Ridgway GL. (1999) Evaluation of microbicidal activity of a new disinfectant, Sterilox 2500, against *Clostridim difficile* spores, *Helicobacter pylori*, vancomycin-resistant enterococcus species, *Candida albicans* and several mycobacterium species. *Journal of Hospital Infection* **41**, 101–105.

Suller MT, Russell AD. (1999) Antibiotic and biocide resistance in methicillin-resistant *Staphylococcus aureus* and vancomycin-resistant enterococcus. *Journal of Hospital Infection* **43**, 281–291.

Taylor DM. (2003) Transmissible degenerative encephalopathies: inactivation of the unconventional causal agents. In: Fraise AP, Lambert PA, Maillard J-Y, eds. *Principles and Practice of Disinfection, Preservation and Sterilization*, 4th edn. Blackwell Science, Oxford. ISBN: 1405101997.

Tyler R, Ayliffe GAJ, Bradley CR. (1990) Virucidal activity of disinfectants: studies with the poliovirus. *Journal of Hospital Infection* **15**, 339–345.

Wilcox MH, Fawley WN, Wigglesworth N, Parnell P, Verity P, Freeman J. (2003) Comparison of the effect of detergent versus hypochlorite cleaning on environmental contamination and incidence of *Clostridium difficile* infection. *Journal of Hospital Infection* **54**, 109–114.

## Further reading

Ayliffe GAJ. (2001) Control of *Staphylococcus aureus* and enterococcal infections. In: Block SS, ed. *Disinfection, Sterilization and Preservation*, 5th edn. Lippincott, Williams & Wilkins, Philadelphia. ISBN: 0683307401.

Fraise AP, Lambert P, Maillard J-Y, eds. (2003) *Russell, Hugo & Ayliffe's Principles and Practice of Disinfection, Preservation and Sterilization*, 4th edn. Blackwell Science, Oxford. ISBN: 1405101997.

Muto CA, Jernigan JA, Ostrowsky BE, Richet HM, Jarvis WR, Boyce JM, Farr BM. (2003) SHEA guideline for preventing nosocomial transmission of multi-drug resistant strains of *Staphylococcus aureus* and enterococcus. *Infection Control and Hospital Epidemiology* **24**, 362–386.

NHS Estates Agency. (1994) *Health technical memorandum 2040. The control of legionellae in healthcare premises: a code of practice. Good practice guide.* NHS Estates, Leeds. ISBN: 0113216831.

NHS Estates Agency. (1994) *Health technical memorandum 2040. The control of legionellae in healthcare premises: a code of practice. Operational management.* NHS Estates, Leeds. ISBN: 0113216823.

NHS Estates Agency. (1994) *Health technical memorandum 2040. The control of legionellae in healthcare premises: a code of practice. Validation and verification.* NHS Estates, Leeds. ISBN: 0113216815.

NHS Estates Agency. (1994) *Health technical memorandum 2040. The control of legionellae in healthcare premises: a code of practice. Management policy.* NHS Estates, Leeds. ISBN: 0113216807.

NHS Estates Agency. (1994) *Health technical memorandum 2040. The control of legionellae in healthcare premises: a code of practice. Design considerations.* NHS Estates, Leeds. ISBN: 0113216793.

NHS Estates Agency. (1995) *Health technical memorandum 2027. Hot and cold water supply, storage and mains services: Operational management.* NHS Estates, Leeds. ISBN: 0113221797.

NHS Estates Agency. (1995) *Health technical memorandum 2027. Hot and cold water supply, storage and mains services: Validation and verification.* NHS Estates, Leeds. ISBN: 0113221789.

NHS Estates Agency. (1995) *Health technical memorandum 2027. Hot and cold water supply, storage and mains services: Design considerations.* NHS Estates, Leeds. ISBN: 0113221770.

NHS Estates Agency. (1995) *Health technical memorandum 2027. Hot and cold water supply, storage and mains services: Management policy.* NHS Estates, Leeds. ISBN: 0113221762.

Working Party of the British Society of Antimicrobial Chemotherapy, the Hospital Infection Society and the Infection Control Nurses Association. (1998) Revised guidelines for the control of methicillin-resistant *Staphylococcus aureus* infection in hospitals. *Journal of Hospital Infection* **39**, 253–290.

# 6 Cleaning and disinfection of the environment

## Wards and operating theatres

Floors and other inanimate surfaces that are physically clean and dry are usually of minor relevance in the spread of endemic infection. Most of the organisms on these surfaces are normal skin flora and aerobic spore-bearing organisms and are unlikely to be an infection hazard to most patients; the skin flora is mainly disseminated on skin scales which are not easily resuspended after settling.

Washing the floor or other horizontal surface with a detergent will remove about 80% of microorganisms, whereas disinfectants will kill or remove about 90–95%. However, in a busy ward, recontamination of the floor after washing or disinfection is rapid and bacterial counts may reach precleaning levels in 1 or 2 hours irrespective of whether a detergent or disinfectant was used (Ayliffe et al., 1966, 1967). This indicates that routine disinfection has little advantage over routine cleaning with detergent in most contexts and has been confirmed in other studies (Dharan et al., 1999).

Most existing clinical studies confirm that routine disinfection of surfaces does not influence the infection rate (Daschner et al., 1980; Danforth et al., 1987), although some workers still believe that the routine use of low-level disinfectants, although of unproven value, is inexpensive and reasonable (Rutala & Weber, 2001). Fogging unoccupied patient areas with disinfectants may provide superficial disinfection but is unproven in respect of infection control.

There is some uncertainty about the possible role of the environment in the spread of some organisms which survive well in the environment, such as C. difficile, MRSA, multiresistant Acinetobacter and VRE (Muto et al., 2003; see also Chapter 5). Routine disinfection or terminal disinfection may be recommended by the infection control team if there is a particular risk in specific areas.

Wet surfaces and equipment are more likely to encourage the growth and spread of potential pathogens, especially opportunist Gram-negative bacilli, and may require disinfection depending on the risk. This applies particularly to cleaning equipment, such as the thermal disinfection of mopheads.

A clean environment is necessary to provide a background to acceptable standards of hygiene, as well as for maintaining the confidence and morale of patients, staff and visitors. Floors and surfaces of wards should be cleaned at least daily, or more frequently in busy units, if soiling is excessive or during outbreaks of infection.

Floors and surfaces of operating theatres should be cleaned at the end of each session. Disinfectants are not usually required, apart from the removal of body fluid spillage, which should occur as soon after the spill as is practicable and not wait until the end of the session. Disinfection of relevant surfaces may sometimes be advised after an operation on an infectious patient. Flooring can be rinsed weekly with water to remove residual detergent or disinfectant to maintain antistatic properties, but this is rarely required.

Walls and ceilings are rarely heavily contaminated and do not act as dispersion sources for contamination (Ayliffe *et al.*, 1967). Cleaning once a year should be adequate in wards and two to four times a year in operating theatres.

## Terminal disinfection

It may be considered necessary to disinfect an isolation room or area following the discharge of a patient infected or colonized with a pathogen transmissible via the environment. Examples of such pathogens are MRSA, VRE, multiresistant *Acinetobacter* and norovirus; others may be specified by the infection control team. Terminal disinfection should include all surfaces that may become contaminated and that are capable of transferring that contamination to a susceptible patient. This will include, amongst other items: floors, mattresses, bed-frames, curtains, patient transfer equipment (hoists and slides), bedside equipment and leads, equipment supports, thermometers, stethoscopes etc. It will not normally include walls and ceilings unless obviously contaminated. For most environmental surfaces, any physical soiling and spillage should be removed and they should then be disinfected with a chlorine-based disinfectant (normally either sodium hypochlorite or NaDCC) at 1000 ppm av Cl where corrosion will not present a problem; a clear soluble phenolic at 1–2% is an alternative. Medical equipment can be wiped with 70% alcohol, after removal of visible soiling. Fabrics should be laundered.

Terminal disinfection of a room should be carried out by specially trained staff. In many hospitals, different categories of staff will have responsibility for disinfecting different items (e.g. the environment such as floors and bed-frames will be disinfected by cleaners, equipment will be disinfected by either nurses, operating department practitioners, medical physics technicians or estates department staff). It is important that all items to be disinfected are allocated to a group of staff, that each individual is aware of their responsibilities and that their activity is coordinated.

## Carpets

There is no good evidence that carpets are associated with an increased infection risk, but care is necessary in deciding on appropriate areas for carpeting. Factors other than infection require consideration, e.g. smell, appearance, comfort, and the likelihood of spillage and staining (Collins, 1979). Carpets in clinical areas associated with frequent or excessive contamination with blood or body fluids (surgical and obstetric) or with food or excreta (units for the mentally handicapped) may be difficult to maintain and avoidance of carpets should be considered. Washable floor surfaces are also advised in isolation rooms and wards.

If carpets are used in clinical areas, they should be washable and quick drying, have a waterproof backing and, if possible, should not be damaged by commonly used disinfectants. Carpets should be vacuum cleaned daily and wet cleaned as necessary, preferably with a steam cleaner. Adequate routine maintenance is important since unpleasant smells or unsightly staining are the main reasons for removal of carpets from wards.

## Body fluid spillage

Spillage should be removed as soon as possible and the area washed with detergent and dried. If spillage is from a known or suspected infected patient it should be removed with a disinfectant, e.g. a chlorine-based agent. If the disinfectant is likely to damage the contaminated surface, such as a carpet, a detergent alone can be used or a disinfectant which does not damage the surface. It is common practice to treat all blood or body fluids as an infection hazard and to remove after applying a disinfectant. We would agree that all spillage should be treated with care and gloves should be worn by the operator, but the value of routine disinfection in blocking infection transmission has not been determined. Some centres may prefer to use a risk assessment approach in deciding what precautions are to be adopted in which instances. Routine disinfection may only be necessary for blood or blood-stained body fluids in areas of significant blood-borne virus infection and in high-risk departments such as accident and emergency and drug dependency units. Small amounts of spillage can be decontaminated before cleaning either with a powder or granules of a chlorine-based agent or peroxygen compound added to an equal volume of the spillage, or with liquid hypochlorite (10 000 ppm av Cl) poured over a paper towel covering the spill. The blood/disinfectant mixture should then be removed safely with paper towels after a short interval (e.g. 1–2 minutes) and the surface wiped with a moistened single-use cloth or paper towel. Larger volumes of body fluid spill should be immobilized either with a disinfectant powder or with absorbent paper towels which are then overlaid with large volumes of a chlorine-based agent (10 000 ppm av Cl). Care should be taken when using chlorine-based compounds in the form of NaDCC, since hazardous quantities of chlorine gas can be released on contact with comparatively mild acids, including some unusually acidic urine spills, particularly if present in large volumes, or dilute acidic cleaning agents. The main hazard of a spill is to the individual clearing it up; they are the most likely to become contaminated. Chemical disinfection is not a process with high quality assurance and infectious agents may survive in a spill treated with disinfectant, particularly if there are dried or clotted areas in it. Gloves should be worn when cleaning up infectious spillage and discarded with any solid blood/powder mixtures and paper towels as clinical waste. Plastic aprons should also be worn if large amounts of spillage are to be removed. Any mops and buckets used should be disinfected after removal of spillage. Thorough cleaning of the surface and wearing of gloves is more important in preventing infection than the use of a disinfectant in the removal of spillage.

## Baths and washbasins

Thoroughly cleaning baths with a detergent after use is usually sufficient. Disinfection of baths and taps may be advisable during outbreaks of infection and following use by infected patients. A non-abrasive, chlorine-based powder or cream is commonly recommended, but a solution of chlorine-based agent with a compatible detergent is a possible alternative.

Antiseptic solutions, e.g. triclosan as *Ster-Zac* bath additive, may be added to the bathwater of patients with infected lesions to reduce the contamination of the water and reduce deposition of organisms on the surface of the bath. Cleaning of bath and taps is still necessary after an antiseptic bath additive has been used.

Washbasins and taps should be cleaned at least daily. Heated sink-traps are of doubtful value in reducing cross-infection.

## Toilets and drains

The toilet seat and handle should be kept clean and washed at least daily; more frequent cleaning and possibly disinfection may be required during outbreaks of infection. A chlorine-based agent or clear soluble phenolic solution may be used, but should be rinsed off the seat before use by the next patient. Toilet pans and sink outlets should be regularly cleaned, but disinfection of pans and pouring disinfectants into drains is of doubtful value.

## Washing bowls

Patient washing bowls should be washed, dried and stored inverted. If used by infected patients, bowls should be washed with a chlorine-based agent or phenolic and then thoroughly rinsed, dried and stored inverted, which allows water remnants to drain by gravity. An individual bowl for each patient may be desirable in high-risk units, e.g. intensive therapy, when it is then terminally disinfected before use by another patient.

## Mattresses

Mattresses should have impermeable covers, which should be inspected regularly to verify that they are intact. They should be cleaned with detergent solutions and dried after patient discharge. If a patient has, or was suspected of having, an infection that may be transmissible, the mattress cover should be disinfected with a chlorine-based agent at 1000 ppm av Cl. Phenolic or alcohol-based disinfectants can damage mattress covers (Department of Health, 1991); compatibility of a particular make of mattress cover should be established via the supplier.

Pneumatic pressure-relieving mattresses ('low air loss' mattresses) should be decontaminated by heat or chemicals in a washing cycle conforming to current UK guidance given in the 'Laundry' section of this chapter (NHS Executive, 1995). This is usually best accomplished by a specialist centre. Many of the companies that offer these mattresses on a rental basis also provide a decontamination service for them. Infection control teams should investigate the adequacy of the decontamination services used by their hospital.

## Kitchens

Prevention of infection from food is achieved mainly by using good hygienic practice, e.g. adequate cooking, cleaning and use of dedicated food preparation surfaces, maintenance of correct refrigeration temperatures and heat disinfection of contaminated utensils and correct storage of foods, rather than by use of chemical disinfectants. If thermal disinfection is required, dish-washing machines should give a final rinse temperature of at least 80°C for 1 minute or another appropriate temperature and time combination to ensure disinfection of the load. In the absence of a machine, thorough cleaning, rinsing and drying is adequate for general wards, but single-use crockery and cutlery may be required for patients with untreated tuberculosis, salmonellosis and some other infectious diseases, if a suitable washing machine is not available.

Disinfectants should only be used in special circumstances on advice from the microbiologist. Disinfectants suitable for kitchen use are chlorine-based agents (120–200 ppm av Cl) or, where these might cause corrosion, quaternary ammonium compounds. Other disinfectants may also be considered, but their microbicidal spectrum, corrosivity, safety and taint-imparting properties must be considered. Phenolic disinfectants should not be used in kitchens as they may taint food even at very low concentrations. Surfaces to which disinfectants are applied should previously have been cleaned. Good handwashing with non-microbicidal agents will remove contamination acquired by touch, and handwashing agents with disinfectants (usually chlorhexidine, povidone-iodine or triclosan) are rarely necessary and should only be used on advice from the infection control team. Nail brushes should be avoided if possible since they damage the skin, but if used, should be regularly disinfected by heat.

## Cleaning equipment

Although not a major source or route of infection, cleaning equipment should be kept clean and stored dry. Vacuum cleaners should be fitted with high-efficiency filters on their exhausts to avoid the redispersion of previously settled contamination. These filters must be replaced when blocked. Dust-attracting mops reduce the dispersal of dust, provided that the mop-heads are changed regularly (e.g. every 2 days or following the manufacturer's instructions). Brooms raise dust and so should not be used.

Wet floor mops should be rinsed after use and dried. They should be regularly thermally disinfected in a washing machine, followed by thorough drying. The normal frequency for this is weekly in ordinary clinical areas and daily in operating theatres and high-risk areas. Chemical disinfection, in a 1000 ppm av Cl chlorine-based disinfectant or a phenolic solution for 30 minutes after preliminary cleaning, is inferior to thermal disinfection and thorough drying. Prolonged storage in a phenolic solution is inadvisable as disinfectant-resistant Gram-negative bacilli may be selected and phenolic solutions may be partially inactivated by plastic mop-heads. Ensuring the mop-head is dry plays a key role in reducing the level of contamination. Single-use mop-heads can be used. Mop buckets should be cleaned and stored inverted. Scrubbing machines should be designed so that tanks can be completely emptied, cleaned and dried.

## Laundry

Fabrics used in healthcare should, wherever possible, be heat disinfected between uses. Current UK guidance (NHS Executive, 1995) is that wash cycles should maintain 65°C for at least 10 minutes or 71°C for at least 3 minutes. Higher temperatures and longer times are acceptable if tolerated by the fabrics. The majority of fabrics ('used' and 'soiled' categories) can be presorted into washing/drying types and loaded into batch continuous washing machines ('tunnel washers'). If the linen constitutes an infectious hazard to laundry staff on sorting ('infected' category), i.e. contaminated with salmonella, shigella, norovirus, etc., it should be carefully loaded into washer extractors without prior sorting and then be subject to a wash with the same thermal disinfection parameters as 'used' and 'soiled' linen receive.

Fabrics that cannot withstand thermal disinfection ('thermolabile') should be put through a wash cycle that provides good dilution and adds a chlorine-based disinfectant to the penultimate rinse to achieve 150 ppm av Cl with a contact time of at least 5 minutes. (The penultimate rinse was chosen as nearly all organic matter and bioburden will have been removed in the wash and early rinse phases, allowing a low disinfectant concentration to be effective. The subsequent rinse will remove the chlorine-based agent, and its smell, from the fabrics.) Use of thermolabile fabrics in healthcare should be kept to a minimum.

The use of domestic washing machines on wards should not be encouraged. However, where ward staff would otherwise wash items by hand in sinks and then air-dry them in unsuitable conditions rather than send them to a laundry, it is safer to allow wards to use washing machines and tumble dryers, provided they are adequately maintained. Fabrics should be washed at the maximum temperature they will tolerate in high-dilution wash cycles and then dried thoroughly. Staff should be trained to use the machines and simple instructions should be clearly displayed by the machines. Advice from the local infection control team should be sought on the safety of using these machines during outbreaks of infection.

# References

Ayliffe GAJ, Collins BJ, Lowbury EJL. (1966) Cleaning and disinfection of hospital floors. *British Medical Journal* **2**, 442–445.

Ayliffe GAJ, Collins BJ, Lowbury EJL. (1967) Ward floors and other surfaces as reservoirs of hospital infection. *Journal of Hygiene (London)* **65**, 515–536.

Collins BJ. (1979) How to have carpeted luxury. *Health and Social Services Journal* (Suppl) 28 September.

Danforth D, Nicoll LE, Hume K, Alfieri N, Sims H. (1987) Nosocomial infections on nursing units with floors cleaned with a disinfectant compared with detergent. *Journal of Hospital Infection* **10**, 229–235.

Daschner F, Rabbenstein G, Langmaack GRH. (1980) Surface contamination in the control of hospital infections: comparison of different methods. *Deutsche Medizinische Wochenschrift* **105**, 325–329.

Department of Health. (1991) *Safety Action Bulletin: Hospital mattress assemblies; care and cleaning*. SAB(91)65. Department of Health, London.

Dharan S, Mouruga P, Copin P, Bessemer G, Tschanz B, Pittet D. (1999) Routine disinfection of patients' environmental surfaces. Myth or reality? *Journal of Hospital Infection* **42**, 113–116.

Muto CA, Jernigan JA, Ostrowsky BE, Richet HM, Jarvis WR, Boyce JM, Farr BM. (2003) SHEA guideline for preventing nosocomial transmission of multi-drug resistant strains of *Staphylococcus aureus* and enterococcus. *Infection Control and Hospital Epidemiology* **24**, 362–386.

NHS Executive. (1995) *Health Service Guidelines: Hospital laundry arrangements for used and infected linen*. HSG(95)18. Department of Health, London.

Rutala WA, Weber DJ. (2001) Surface disinfection: should we do it ? *Journal of Hospital Infection* **48** (Suppl. A), S64–S68.

# Further reading

Ayliffe GAJ, Babb JR, Taylor LJ. (1999) *Hospital-Acquired Infection. Principles and Prevention*, 3rd edn. Butterworth Heinemann, Oxford. ISBN: 0750621052.

Ayliffe GAJ, Fraise AP, Geddes AM, Mitchell K, eds. (2000) *Control of Hospital Infection: A Practical Handbook*, 4th edn. Arnold, London. ISBN: 0340759119.

Bradley CR. (2003) Treatment of laundry and clinical waste in hospitals. In: Fraise AP, Lambert P, Maillard J-Y, eds. *Russell, Hugo & Ayliffe's Principles and Practice of Disinfection, Preservation and Sterilization*, 4th edn. Blackwell Science, Oxford. ISBN: 1405101997.

Hoffman PN. (1993) Cleaning and disinfection. In: Hobbs BC, Roberts D, eds. *Food Poisoning and Food Hygiene*, 6th edn. Arnold, London. ISBN: 034053740.

Maki DG, Alvarado CJ, Hassemer CA, Zilz MA. (1982) Relation of the inanimate environment to endemic nosocomial infections. *New England Journal of Medicine* **307**, 1562–1566.

# 7 Disinfection of the skin and mucous membranes

## Introduction

In the context of skin contamination and decontamination, microorganisms on the skin can be classified as 'resident' or 'transients'. The 'resident' flora, mainly coagulase-negative staphylococci, micrococci and diphtheroids, grow on the surface of the skin and in the pores and follicles beneath the surface. The resident microflora are usually of low pathogenicity. Those located below the skin surface cannot be removed by washing or killed by disinfection (Selwyn & Ellis, 1972). They are common causes of infection following implant surgery, such as hip replacements, and at intravascular insertion sites. *Staphylococcus aureus* frequently colonizes the anterior nares and less frequently other areas of skin, such as the perineum.

The 'transient' organisms are those deposited on the skin from the environment, for example by touching a contaminated object. They do not usually grow on the skin and will either die, or be removed by contact or washing. As they are usually present only on the surface of the skin, they can be removed readily by washing or disinfection. The transient flora are responsible for most hospital cross-infection and include, amongst others, *Staph. aureus, Pseudomonas aeruginosa*, salmonellae, other Gram-negative bacilli and viruses. *Staph. aureus* and *Klebsiella* spp. may occasionally survive and grow on the skin for several days or longer and are often described as 'temporary residents'. *Acinetobacter* spp. are the only Gram-negative bacilli that colonize certain areas of skin and can be described as true residents; however, if acquired by touch, they will behave as transients. *Staph. aureus* and Gram-negative bacilli may colonize damaged or eczematous skin.

## Handwashing and disinfection

The hands of healthcare workers with patient contact are one of the main vehicles of cross-infection, and washing or disinfecting hands is probably the most important measure for preventing the spread of such infection.

It is of greater importance in high-risk units and during outbreaks of infection. Physical removal of transient contaminants by washing with soap or detergent and water is a very effective means of infection control.

• Failure to wash or disinfect the hands at the right time is one of the major problems of infection control and continuing education of staff to produce sustained compliance is necessary.
• Washing or disinfecting hands thoroughly at the right time is more important than the agent used or the length of time of application.

Optimal times of application of antiseptics are uncertain, but the times suggested below are based on laboratory experiments or are accepted in clinical practice in the UK (Table 5). Times recommended by

**Table 5:** Summary of hand cleansing categories.

|  | Routine handwash | Hygienic hand disinfection | Surgical hand disinfection |
|---|---|---|---|
| WHY | Use soap or detergent to remove transient microorganisms. Hygienic hand disinfection with alcohol can be a convenient alternative | Use antiseptics (detergent–disinfectant mixtures or alcoholic handrubs) to remove or destroy high levels of transient microorganisms | Use antiseptics (detergent–disinfectant mixtures or alcoholic handrubs) to remove or destroy transient microorganisms and substantially reduce resident microorganisms. A prolonged effect is required |
| HOW | A thorough wash with a soap or detergent or rubbing a small volume of alcohol into the hands to evaporation | A thorough wash for 15–30 s with antiseptic soap or detergent. Alternatively apply an alcohol handrub to disinfect clean hands | Apply antiseptic detergent to hands and forearms for a minimum of 2 min. Alternatively, clean hands with soap and water and apply two or more applications of an alcohol antiseptic handrub |
| WHEN | Before and after all patient contacts | During outbreaks of infection, in high-risk areas, when contact with infectious material is likely or on the advice of the infection control team | Prior to gloving for surgery or invasive procedures or on the advice of the infection control team. |

manufacturers for their own products are usually satisfactory but should be based on laboratory studies.

It is important that any agent used for handwashing or disinfection should be acceptable to users, i.e. it should be easy and pleasant to use and must not damage the skin on repeated use. Provision of unacceptable agents will decrease compliance with hand hygiene.

Handwashing or disinfection may be classified as routine, hygienic or surgical.

## Routine handwashing

Routine handwashing is effective in removing most transient organisms and can be used as a routine procedure in healthcare establishments. This includes the following occasions:

- removing physical dirt (including blood, excretions, secretions or discharges from lesions);
- on arriving in and leaving a patient area;
- after using the toilet;
- before preparing or handling food or medicines;
- before and after routine patient contact; and
- after bedmaking or bedbathing.

### *Procedure*

- Wet hands under running water and add sufficient liquid soap or detergent to cupped hands to obtain a good lather.
- Wash hands for 15–20 seconds without adding more water.
- Ensure all areas of hands are covered during the process, paying special attention to the tips of the fingers and the thumbs (see Fig. 1) (Ayliffe *et al.*, 1978; Taylor, 1978).
- Rinse thoroughly under running water and dry with a disposable towel.

## Hygienic hand disinfection

Preparations of detergent containing an antiseptic, such as 4% chlorhexidine, 0.75% povidone-iodine or 1% triclosan or alcohol solutions are commonly used.

- Products used for hygienic handwashing should conform to the standard EN 1499 (British Standards Institution, 1997a) and to EN 1500 (British Standards Institution, 1997b) for hygienic handrubs.

### *Hygienic hand disinfection with aqueous formulations*

Transient organisms are more effectively removed or destroyed with a detergent–disinfectant mixture than with a soap or detergent and

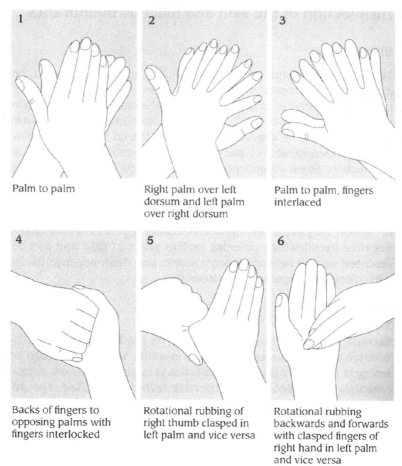

Figure 1: Hand washing and disinfection technique. Apply 3–5 mL of the formulation to the cupped hands and carry out steps 1–6 one or more times using the following procedure. Each step consists of three strokes (routine or hygienic hand-disinfection) or five strokes (surgical hand-disinfection) backwards and forwards. (See also Ayliffe GAJ, *et al.*, 1978.)

water wash. Whilst a residual microbicidal effect may be obtained from some detergent–disinfectant mixtures, the practical value of this against transient contamination acquired following disinfection is doubtful and should not be relied upon as a substitute for performing a hygienic hand-wash every time it is required.

Hygienic handwashing is frequently used for the following:

- contact with contaminated secretions or excretions or other infectious materials;
- contact with infected or colonized patients or their immediate surroundings;
- in high-risk units such as intensive care and burns;
- on entering protective isolation units and leaving source isolation units;
- before aseptic procedures, e.g. dressing techniques and minor invasive procedures.

### Procedure

- Hands are moistened.
- 3–5 ml of the antiseptic detergent (or as recommended by the manufacturer) are added to the cupped hands and applied to all areas for 15–20 seconds as described for routine handwashing (see Fig. 1).
- Hands are rinsed thoroughly and dried with a paper towel.

### Hygienic hand disinfection with alcohol formulations

Alcohol handrubs, as either liquid or gelled products, are used for hygienic hand disinfection. They can also be used as an alternative to routine handwashing, where there is no visible soiling, for all ward procedures and patient contacts. They are often more convenient than handwashing and can be particularly useful if handwash basins are not readily available. Dispensers for alcohol handrubs can be fitted by handwashing sinks and can also be placed beside each bed or carried around by each healthcare worker. They are generally more effective in killing transient organisms than aqueous detergent–disinfectant solutions and can be used before aseptic procedures, in high-risk units or after handling contaminated sites or materials. Their use is particularly valuable during outbreaks of infection, especially of highly virulent or antibiotic-resistant organisms (Rotter, 1984; Ayliffe *et al.*, 1988; Pittet *et al.*, 2000). Ethanol at 70% or isopropanol at 60% with an emollient to prevent drying of skin (e.g. 1% glycerol), with or without an added antiseptic (usually chlorhexidine or triclosan), are commonly used. Higher concentrations of alcohol than these tend to be less effective against bacteria. A residual effect on the hands may be obtained if an antiseptic is added to the alcohol, but the practical value of this against transient contamination acquired following disinfection is doubtful and should not be relied upon as a substitute for performing hygienic disinfection every time it is required. Alcohol, especially isopropanol, may not be effective against non-enveloped viruses due to the short exposure time of the agent on the hands and the inherent resistance of the virus (Davies *et al.*, 1993). Ethanol at 85–90% is generally more effective than at 60–70% against these agents, but washing hands is preferable if contamination with these viruses is possible. Ethanol at 70% is effective, however, against rotaviruses (Bellamy *et al.*, 1993). Alcohols have no activity against bacterial spores; handwashing is more appropriate than alcohol handrubs during outbreaks of infection with spore-forming organisms, such as *Clostridium difficile*.

- Alcohol solutions are flammable (and potentially hazardous, particularly when large amounts are stored).
- Alcohols do not penetrate organic matter; visibly soiled hands should be decontaminated by washing.
- Products used for hygienic hand disinfection should conform to the standard EN 1500 (British Standards Institution, 1997b).

### Procedure
- A volume of 2–3 ml (or as recommended by manufacturer) of the alcoholic solution or gel is applied to the cupped hands and rubbed to dryness, covering all surfaces of the hands.
- Hands should be wet with alcohol for about 15 seconds.
- More alcohol can be applied if hands dry out too quickly.

## Surgical hand disinfection
Surgical hand disinfection requires the removal or killing of transients and a substantial reduction in and a suppression of regrowth of the resident microflora for the duration of the surgical procedure (Lowbury *et al.*, 1963; Newsom, 1999). As glove punctures during surgery are not uncommon, a residual disinfectant effect is of value in maintaining low bacterial levels during the operation. Rings with stones and other jewellery are removed and the nails are cleaned with a manicure stick if required, and scrubbed with a sterile brush or sponge before the first operation of the day. The use of a brush should be discontinued before subsequent operations since the damage caused to the skin increases the risk of colonization with pathogenic bacteria.

### Surgical hand disinfection with aqueous formulations
Similar antiseptic detergents are used as for hygiene handwashing, detailed above, but with a longer exposure time.

## Procedure

- Hands are moistened with water and 3–5 ml (or as recommended by the manufacturer) of the antiseptic detergent applied thoroughly to the hands and forearms.
- Washing without rinsing continues for 2–3 minutes. All areas of hands and forearms should be adequately covered; more antiseptic can be added if required.
- Hands and forearms are thoroughly rinsed in running water and dried with a disposable or sterilized towel.

### Surgical hand disinfection with alcohol formulations

Alcohol solutions (60–70% ethanol or isopropanol) with an emollient and with or without an added antiseptic as recommended for hygienic hand disinfection (above) are used, but using larger volumes and longer exposure times than for hygienic hand disinfection (Lowbury *et al.*, 1974; Rotter, 2003). Based on laboratory studies, they are microbiologically more effective than the traditional surgical scrub, although it remains uncertain whether they are more clinically effective.

### Procedure

- Before the first procedure, wash hands with liquid soap or detergent.
- An alcohol–antiseptic mixture, about 5 ml, is applied to hands and forearms.
- The solution is thoroughly rubbed into hands and forearms.
- The alcohol solution is rubbed to dryness.
- The procedure is repeated with a second 5-ml volume of alcohol–antiseptic.

If allergy to an antiseptic occurs, a preliminary bland soap and water wash, followed by drying, followed by an alcohol rub without antiseptic is acceptable. Alcoholic solutions even without an added antiseptic have a greater immediate and prolonged effect than an antiseptic detergent, but are rarely used without an added antiseptic.

Some surgeons may prefer to wash and scrub their hands initially with an antiseptic detergent at the beginning of the operating session and continue with a single alcohol rub (3 ml) for subsequent operations or if a glove is punctured (Selwyn & Ellis, 1972). If there is visible blood contamination of the hand, this should be washed off, the hands dried and then the alcohol applied. (Alcohols do not penetrate proteinaceous matter.)

## User acceptability

Any preparation used for handwashing or disinfection must be acceptable to the user and not damage the skin on repeated use (Scott *et al.*, 1991; Kownatzki, 2003). If the preparation is not accepted by staff it will not be used. Damaged skin will also increase the number of resident organisms and may become heavily colonized with *Staph. aureus*. Allergic reactions may occur with specific antiseptics or detergents and alternatives should be tried. Maintaining good skin condition is particularly necessary for staff carrying out many handwashes during the day, and a good quality hand cream, compatible with any antiseptic used, should be applied as required. A personal dispenser is preferred as communal jars of hand cream may become contaminated.

Alcoholic solutions with an emollient are usually less irritant than antiseptic detergents, but staff sensitive to detergents may have to use a bland soap or detergent preparation for handwashing. A trial of acceptability should be introduced with each new preparation.

## Variations in effectiveness of similar preparations

Preparations with the same concentration of the same active ingredient can behave differently due to other factors such as the method of dispensing, interference from the detergent or other components of the formulation. Each preparation should be tested for efficacy (Babb *et al.*, 1991).

## Drying hands after washing

Thorough drying is important since organisms are more readily transferred from wet hands. Drying with a paper towel also removes further organisms remaining on the skin after washing and rinsing. Drying of hands is also important, especially during the winter, to avoid possible chapping. Good-quality paper towels with good drying properties are advised in clinical areas. Sterile hand towels should be used in the operating theatre.

Hot air hand dryers may be preferred in non-clinical areas such as toilets but they are often noisy and as they are slower than paper towels, the inconvenience may not encourage handwashing. Roller towels may be used in non-clinical areas, but they could transfer contamination between users if not changed immediately a roll is finished.

# Gloves

Handwashing or disinfection will not necessarily remove all the transient organisms, particularly if microbial contamination is heavy. In addition to handwashing, non-sterile gloves should be worn when handling wound dressings, emptying urinary drainage bags, and handling bedpans or bedding contaminated with faeces, particularly during outbreaks of enteric virus infection. Gloves are usually worn when handling blood or other body fluids to reduce risks from unrecognized infections.

Handwashing is still recommended after removal of gloves as glove punctures can be frequent and contamination can pass through onto the hands, and there is the possibility of contaminating hands if glove removal technique is poor. Organisms are readily removed from the surface of gloves, but washing gloved hands is undesirable as the lack of tactile feedback can lead to a less effective washing technique and any contamination that has passed through small punctures in the gloves will be left in contact with the skin. Sterile gloves are worn for operative procedures, providing an additional barrier to hand disinfection.

Allergy to the latex in gloves may occur and is a serious condition. Latex proteins can be carried on starch granules and can cause serious respiratory symptoms and eczema. There should be a local policy on prevention of latex allergies. Powder-free and hypoallergenic latex gloves should be used. Gloves made from non-latex materials should be available if required.

# Preoperative disinfection of the patient's skin

As for surgical scrubs, agents used for preoperative disinfection of the patient's skin should be active against both the 'transient' and 'resident flora', but the effect should last for the days that the wound will be covered, rather than the hours that a surgeon's hands would be gloved. The final preparation to be used on the operation site should be rapidly acting and have a prolonged residual effect. Alcoholic solutions of 0.5% chlorhexidine, povidone-iodine containing 1% available iodine or 0.5% triclosan are most frequently used (Davies *et al.*, 1978; Newsom, 1999). Iodine (not as povidone-iodine) in 70% ethanol can also be used, but it can give rise to skin reactions.

### Procedure
Apply the antiseptic to the operation site with friction using gauze or the operating gloved hand for at least 2–3 minutes. The area covered should

extend well beyond the operation site. If a gloved hand is used to apply the antiseptic, a second glove should be worn over the operating glove and removed when the preparation of the operation site is complete. Alcoholic solutions are highly flammable and must be allowed to dry thoroughly before the operation. They should be applied such that pooling beneath the patient does not occur, especially if diathermy or electocautery is to be used (Medical Devices Agency, 2000). Severe burns to patients undergoing surgery have resulted from the ignition of alcohol solutions left behind after skin preparation.

## Longer-term preoperative patient skin disinfection

A high cumulative reduction in 'residents' can be obtained by repeated applications of aqueous chlorhexidine or triclosan, but a thorough application of an alcoholic solution to the operation site is as, or more, effective (Lilly et al., 1979). The effect of preoperative bathing or showering on infection rates remains controversial. A single bath preoperatively with chlorhexidine detergent is unlikely to reduce the risk of infection (Ayliffe et al., 1983) but studies on repeated bathing have shown variable results (Hayek et al., 1987; Rotter et al., 1988). The effect of repeated bathing is likely to be marginal if the skin of the operation site is well prepared at operation, but nevertheless antiseptic baths are often recommended before cardiovascular or prosthetic surgery. If antiseptic bathing or showering is used the solution should be thoroughly applied to all areas of the moistened skin and then rinsed off.

## Bacterial spores on skin

Ingrained dirt on the skin (e.g. the hands of gardeners) or dried faeces on the skin of incontinent patients may be contaminated with clostridial spores. Removal by washing with detergents or grease solvent gels, followed by an application of 1% aqueous povidone-iodine to the operation site for at least 30 minutes will reduce, but not necessarily eliminate, spores on the skin (Lowbury et al., 1964). Routine methods of skin disinfection are ineffective against bacterial spores. Prophylactic penicillin should be given to all patients at risk from gas gangrene, e.g. lower limb amputations for poor blood supply or diabetic gangrene.

## Preoperative disinfection of mucous membranes

Applications of aqueous solutions of povidone-iodine or chlorhexidine are effective for disinfection of oral mucous membranes, but some dental surgeons consider disinfection to be of doubtful value in the prevention of infection. Alcoholic solutions are more rapid in activity than aqueous but may be rendered ineffective by normal secretions.

A douche with 0.5% povidone-iodine followed by use of a povidone-iodine gel may be used for disinfection of the vaginal mucosa. Obstetric cream containing chlorhexidine is also commonly used, but the effect on clinical infection is uncertain. A 1% chlorhexidine cream instilled into the urethra will disinfect this site before cystoscopy or catheterization.

## Treatment of staphylococcal carriers

It is not necessary to treat nasal carriers of *Staph. aureus* unless the strain is causing infection in the carriers themselves or treatment is required as part of the control of an outbreak. Routine treatment of MRSA carriers has been recommended (Hudson, 1994; Working Party Report, 1998). To treat nasal carriers, an antibacterial cream is applied to the anterior nares three or four times a day for 5–7 days and repeated for a further course if necessary. Two per cent mupirocin in a paraffin base (*Bactroban*) has been shown to be more effective in removing staphylococci than other agents and relapses are less common. However, resistance has been reported, and if possible its use should be restricted to carriers of MRSA and pro-longed use avoided. For removal of methicillin-sensitive or mupirocin-resistant strains, less effective creams or ointments should be considered, e.g. neomycin–chlorhexidine (*Naseptin*), neomycin–bacitracin, povidone-iodine or 1% chlorhexidine. Agents which are useful for treating systemic infections such as gentamicin or fusidic acid should preferably not be used topically since the emergence of resistance could cause problems in treatment of severe infections. Systemic treatment of nasal carriers should be used only in exceptional circumstances. Rifampicin is one of the most effective agents but owing to the rapid emergence of resistance it should always be used in combination with another agent to which the organism is sensitive, such as fusidic acid or ciprofloxacin.

Since nasal and skin carriers are likely to contaminate other areas of skin, they should also wash routinely and bath or shower daily for at least a week with an antiseptic detergent containing chlorhexidine, povidone-iodine or triclosan.

## Treatment of throat carriers

The role of staphylococcal throat carriers in the transmission of infections remains uncertain, but if it is considered of importance spraying the throat with 0.2% chlorhexidine for 3 weeks has been reported as effective (Balfour *et al.*, 1997). Systemic antibiotics as described above may also be used in exceptional circumstances.

## Prevention of staphylococcal colonization in neonates

Selective antibacterial agents have been found useful in preventing colonization of babies with *Staph. aureus*. However, the necessity of applying an antiseptic preparation routinely to all babies in the absence of staphylococcal infection in the unit is of uncertain value and it may be preferable to retain the use of antiseptics only for such problems. Bathing the baby or washing susceptible areas with 4% chlorhexidine–detergent will reduce staphylococcal colonization and is useful during outbreaks. Application of powders containing hexachlorophane (e.g. *Ster-Zac*) or chlorhexidine to the umbilicus (normally the primary site of *Staph. aureus* colonization), groin, buttocks, axillae and lower abdomen also reduces the rate of colonization with *Staph. aureus* whilst allowing normal colonization with coagulase-negative staphylococci (Alder *et al.*, 1980). The selective colonization with Gram-negative bacilli on a moist umbilicus is a possible disadvantage. Bathing or washing with hexachlorophane detergents should be avoided because of potential toxicity.

## References

Alder VG, Burman D, Simpson RA, Fysh J, Gillespie WA. (1980) Comparison of hexachlorophane and chlorhexidine powders in prevention of neonatal infection. *Archives of Disease in Childhood* **55**, 277–280.

Ayliffe GAJ, Babb JR, Quoraishi AH. (1978) A test for hygienic hand disinfection. *Journal of Clinical Pathology* **31**, 923–928.

Ayliffe GA, Noy MF, Babb JR, Davies JG, Jackson J. (1983) A comparison of pre-operative bathing with chlorhexidine–detergent and non-medicated soap in the prevention of wound infection. *Journal of Hospital Infection* **4**, 237–244.

Ayliffe GAJ, Babb JR, Davies JG, Lilly HA. (1988) Hand disinfection: a comparison of various agents in laboratory and ward studies. *Journal of Hospital Infection* **11**, 226–243.

Babb JR, Davies JG, Ayliffe GAJ. (1991) A test procedure for evaluating surgical hand disinfection. *Journal of Hospital Infection* **18** (Suppl. B), 41–49.

Balfour A, Higgins J, Brown M, Gallacher G. (1997) Eradication of throat carriage of methicillin-resistant *Staphylococcus aureus*. *Journal of Hospital Infection* **35**, 320–321.

Bellamy K, Alcock R, Babb JR, Aylitte GAJ. (1993) A test for the assessment of 'hygienic' hand disinfection using rotavirus. *Journal of Hospital Infection* **24**, 201–210.

British Standards Institution (1997a) BS EN 1499:1997. *Chemical disinfectants and antiseptics. Hygienic handwash. Test method and requirements (phase 2/step 2).* British Standards Institution, London.

British Standards Institution (1997b) BS EN 1500:1997. *Chemical disinfectants and antiseptics. Hygienic handrub. Test method and requirements (phase 2/step 2).* British Standards Institution, London.

Davies J, Babb JR, Ayliffe GA, Wilkins MD. (1978) Disinfection of the skin of the abdomen. *British Journal of Surgery* **65**, 855–858.

Davies JG, Babb JR, Bradley CR, Ayliffe GAJ. (1993) Preliminary study of test methods to assess the virucidal activity of skin disinfectants using poliovirus and bacteriophages. *Journal of Hospital Infection* **25**, 125–131.

Hayek LJ, Emerson JM, Gardner AMN. (1987) A placebo-controlled trial of the effect of two preoperative baths or showers with chlorhexidine detergent on postoperative wound infection rates. *Journal of Hospital Infection* **10**, 165–172.

Hudson IRB. (1994) The efficacy of intranasal mupirocin in the prevention of staphylococcal infections: a review of recent experience. *Journal of Hospital Infection* **27**, 81–88.

Kownatzki E. (2003) Hand hygiene and skin health. *Journal of Hospital Infection* **55**, 239–245.

Lilly HA, Lowbury EJL, Wilkins MD. (1979) Limits to progressive reduction of skin bacteria by disinfection. *Journal of Clinical Pathology* **32**, 382–385.

Lowbury EJL, Lilly HA, Bull JP. (1963) Disinfection of the hands: removal of resident flora. *British Medical Journal* **1**, 1251–1256.

Lowbury EJL, Lilly HA, Bull JP. (1964) Methods of disinfection of the hands and operation sites. *British Medical Journal* **2**, 531–536.

Lowbury EJL, Lilly HA, Ayliffe GAJ. (1974) Preoperative disinfection of surgeon's hands: use of alcoholic solutions and effects of gloves on skin flora. *British Medical Journal* **1**, 369–372.

Medical Devices Agency. (2000) *Safety Notice: Use of spirit-based solutions during surgical procedures requiring the use of electrosurgical equipment.* MDA SN2000(17). Medical Devices Agency, London.

Newsom SWB. (1999) Special problems in hospital antisepsis. In: Russell AD, Hugo WB, Ayliffe GAJ, eds. *Principles and Practice of Disinfection, Preservation and Sterilization*, 3rd edn. Blackwell Science, Oxford. ISBN: 0632041943.

Pittet D, Hugonnet S, Harbarth S, Mourouga P, Sauvan V, Touveneau S, Perneger TV. (2000) Effectiveness of a hospital-wide programme to improve compliance with hand hygiene. *Lancet* **356**, 1307–1312.

Rotter ML. (1984) Hygienic hand disinfection. *Infection Control* **5**, 18–22.

Rotter ML. (2003) Special problems in hospital antisepsis. In: Fraise AP, Lambert P, Maillard J-Y, eds. *Russell, Hugo & Ayliffe's Principles and Practice of Disinfection, Preservation and Sterilization*, 4th edn. Blackwell Science, Oxford. ISBN: 1405101997.

Rotter ML, Larsen SO, Cooke EM, Dankert J, Daschner F, Greco D, Gronross P, Jepsen OB, Lystad A, Nystrom B. The European Working Party on Control of Hospital Infections. (1988) A comparison of the effects of preoperative whole-body bathing with detergent alone and with detergent containing chlorhexidine gluconate on the frequency of wound infections after clean surgery. *Journal of Hospital Infection* **11**, 310–320.

Scott D, Barnes A, Lister M, Arkell P. (1991) An evaluation of user acceptability of chlorhexidine handwash formulations. *Journal of Hospital Infection* **18** (Suppl. B), 51–58.

Selwyn S, Ellis H. (1972) Skin bacteria and skin disinfection reconsidered. *British Medical Journal* **1**, 136–140.

Taylor LJ. (1978) An evaluation of handwashing techniques. *Nursing Times* **74**, 54–56; 108–110.

Working Party of the British Society of Antimicrobial Chemotherapy, the Hospital Infection Society and the Infection Control Nurses Association. (1998) Revised guidelines for the control of methicillin-resistant *Staphylococcus aureus* infection in hospitals. *Journal of Hospital Infection* **39**, 253–290.

## Further reading

Ayliffe GAJ, Fraise AP, Geddes AM, Mitchell K, eds. (2000) *Control of Hospital Infection: A Practical Handbook*, 4th edn. Arnold, London. ISBN: 0340759119.

Block SS, ed. (2001) *Disinfection, Sterilization and Preservation*, 5th edn. Lippincott, Williams & Wilkins, Philadelphia. ISBN: 0683307401.

Boyce JM, Pittet D. (2002) Healthcare Infection Control Practices Advisory Committee. Society for Healthcare Epidemiology of America. Association for Professionals in Infection Control. Infectious Diseases Society of America. Hand Hygiene Task Force. Guideline for Hand Hygiene in Health-Care Settings: recommendations of the Healthcare Infection Control Practices Advisory Committee and the HICPAC/SHEA/APIC/IDSA Hand Hygiene Task Force. *Infection Control and Hospital Epidemiology* **23** (12 Suppl.), S3–S40.

Hand Washing Liaison Group. (1999) Handwashing—a modest measure with a big effect. *British Medical Journal* **318**, 686.

Larson EL, Early E, Cloonan P, Sugrue S, Parides M. (2000) An organizational climate intervention associated with increased handwashing and decreased nosocomial infections. *Behavioral Medicine* **26**, 14–22.

Mayhall CG. (2000) *Hospital Epidemiology and Infection Control*. Lippincott, Williams & Wilkins, Philadelphia. ISBN: 0683306081.

Muto CA, Jernigan JA, Ostrowsky BE, Richet HM, Jarvis WR, Boyce JM, Farr BM. (2003) SHEA guideline for preventing nosocomial transmission of multi-drug resistant strains of *Staphylococcus aureus* and enterococcus. *Infection Control and Hospital Epidemiology* **24**, 362–386.

Pellowe CM, Pratt RJ, Harper P, Loveday HP, Robinson N, Jones SRLJ, MacRae ED. (2003) Prevention of healthcare-associated infections in primary and community care. *Journal of Hospital Infection* **55** (Suppl. 2), S5–S127.

Rotter M. (1996) Handwashing and hand disinfection. In: Mayhall CG, ed. *Hospital Epidemiology and Infection Control*. Williams & Wilkins, Baltimore. ISBN: 0683306081.

# 8 Disinfection of medical equipment

A more comprehensive list of items used in healthcare and options for their decontamination is given in the Appendix, p. 93.

## Respiratory equipment

Mechanical ventilators, humidifiers and associated tubing and equipment are frequently contaminated with *Pseudomonas aeruginosa* or other Gram-negative bacilli. Disinfection of a ventilator after use by each patient is unnecessary provided it is protected by bacteria-impermeable filters. If decontamination is required, steam sterilization is preferred as this process has a good quality assurance, although spore-bearing organisms are not a cause of respiratory infection. The smaller ventilators can often be decontaminated with ethylene oxide, if available. The hazards of infection can also be reduced by reducing the amount of condensation in a circuit by the use of heat–moisture exchangers and moisture traps.

The external circuit, and often the humidifiers, can be disinfected in a washer-disinfector which holds items at a minimum of 71°C for 3 minutes, 80°C for 1 minute, 90°C for 12 seconds or another appropriate time/temperature combination. A washer-disinfector adapted to take tubing should be available for treating respiratory equipment. Single-use circuits can be used but can be more expensive.

The external circuit should be changed every 48 hours or between patients. This can be reduced to weekly or between patients if a heat–moisture exchanger is used. Humidifiers can often be decontaminated by increasing the temperature of the water to 70°C or higher. Humidifiers should be cleaned and dried and refilled with sterile water every 48–72 hours. If nebulizers are used, they should be rinsed in alcohol after cleaning if heat disinfection is not possible.

Anaesthetic equipment is mainly contaminated close to the patient (i.e. facemask and proximal part of tubing) and treatment of the machine is rarely necessary. A filter should be included between the patient and machine which should be changed after each patient. A single-use circuit is recommended if the equipment is used on a case of open tuberculosis. The circuit should be replaced at least every session (i.e. 10–12 patients) and treated in a washer-disinfector adapted to take tubing. Replacement of the circuit after every patient is preferable but clean facemasks should always be provided for each patient.

When resources are limited and single-use equipment is too expensive if regularly changed as indicated above, thorough cleaning, immersion in a chlorine-based agent (200 ppm av Cl) and thorough rinsing before reuse is a possible alternative if the items are not damaged by chlorine. Glutaraldehyde is too irritant and should not be used for soaking respiratory equipment.

## Endoscopes

Endoscopes present a substantial challenge with respect to decontamination. They are complex items, comparatively easily damaged and with long, narrow channels that are difficult to gain access to for cleaning and disinfection.

- Their high cost favours rapid methods of decontamination: the faster the turnaround, the fewer instruments will be needed during a session.
- Endoscopes have a variety of materials in their composition and it is impossible to predict if these will be compatible with particular formulations of disinfectant without practical observations. Reliable data on compatibility are vital.
- Chemical disinfectants have to be used safely with respect to staff health; it is preferable to use non-toxic agents, but if hazardous substances are used, effective measures to prevent them harming staff and patients must be in place. Safe alternatives to glutaraldehyde are currently being sought by many endoscope reprocessors in the UK, with many new disinfectant formulations being tried.
- New chemical agents should be used for exposure times as recommended by the manufacturers or by the relevant professional body.
- Efficient cleaning of all channels is vital before any decontamination, both for the efficacy of disinfection and as some chemical agents will coagulate ('fix') proteins onto surfaces, causing lumens to block. Cleaning will inevitably have a manual phase which must be done by trained staff with adequate equipment.
- Accessories used with endoscopes (biopsy forceps etc.) need at least the same quality of decontamination as the endoscopes. Single-use or heat-sterilizable accessories are preferred.

- Automated washer-disinfectors are preferred to manual disinfection but users need to be aware that they may become a source of microbial contamination and subsequent recontamination of processed endoscopes.
- Rinsing to remove disinfectant residues is an important part of the process, but care must be taken not to recontaminate processed endoscopes.

## Operative endoscopes

Operative (invasive) endoscopes (e.g. arthroscopes and laparoscopes) should be sterilized, and many are now approved by their manufacturers as compatible with steam sterilization. Heat sterilization of these items in a sterile supplies department or equivalent is recommended. Ethylene oxide is an alternative method of sterilization, but is not often available for routine use and involves a much longer turnaround time. The newer operative endoscopes are often flexible and will not withstand heat. Suitable automated washer-disinfectors for use with chemical disinfectants are now available, but care should be taken to avoid microbial recontamination on postdisinfection rinsing.

The use of liquid chemical agents in a sporicidal process, such as immersion in 2% glutaraldehyde for 3 hours, is an alternative to heat sterilization but the long time involved is inconvenient and processing has to occur immediately before use as the endoscope can become rapidly contaminated after rinsing. Significant numbers of bacterial spores are unlikely to be present in a well-cleaned endoscope and pathogenic spores are less resistant to glutaraldehyde than those commonly used for test purposes. High-level disinfection (i.e. disinfection without a significant sporicidal action) immediately before use is usually adequate. The minimum effective immersion time in a disinfectant between use of the endoscope in successive patients is generally accepted as 10 minutes in glutaraldehyde, although 20 minutes should be used if activity against *Mycobacterium tuberculosis* is required. Other more rapidly sporicidal disinfectants are now available, such as peracetic acid, chlorine dioxide and superoxidized water. Most of these agents will give sporicidal activity within 10 minutes, but users should establish the recommended contact times from the disinfectant manufacturer. Thorough rinsing with sterile water is important to remove disinfectant residues.

Most rigid cystoscopes are heat tolerant and can be processed by autoclaving. Heat-labile cystoscopes can be adequately treated by thorough cleaning, followed by exposure to glutaraldehyde for a minimum of 10 minutes, or an alternative compatible agent for a time recommended by the manufacturer, in a washer-disinfector. Spore-forming organisms are unlikely to cause urinary tract infections.

All endoscopes and accessories should be thoroughly cleaned following the manufacturer's recommended instructions before immersion, and invasive instruments must be rinsed in sterile water before reuse. Systems are now available for automated irrigation of cleaning solution down the lumens of rigid endoscopes. Bacteria-free water may be acceptable but the microbiological quality of the water must be regularly checked (NHS Estates Agency, 1997).

## Flexible endoscopes

Flexible endoscopes have components that will be affected by high temperatures, so none are currently amenable to steam sterilization or heat disinfection. Use of chemical disinfectants is currently the only practicable option for decontamination.

Flexible endoscopes should be manually cleaned by brushing all accessible channels and flushing them with a detergent solution. This should be followed by an automated disinfection cycle in a washer-disinfector comprising thorough irrigation of all channels (i.e. biopsy, suction, air, water, forceps raiser and auxiliary channels) with detergent, followed by disinfectant, then thorough rinsing. This should be done between patients.

The professional societies in the UK (Cooke *et al.*, 1993; British Thoracic Society Bronchoscopy Guidelines Committee, 2001; British Society of Gastroenterology, 2003) and the Medical Devices Agency (2002) have issued recommendations for decontamination.

### Cleaning of flexible endoscopes

Manual precleaning is recommended even if an automated endoscope washer-disinfector that includes a detergent-flushing stage is used. This should include brushing of all accessible channels and flushing of all channels with a freshly prepared detergent solution. It is important to ensure that the correct size brush is used to ensure contact with all accessible surfaces. The brush itself should be cleaned between uses and must be inspected regularly to ensure it is still sufficiently intact to clean adequately. There is now a move towards single-use brushes to remove the problem of cleaning and inspecting them, and to eliminate the risk of transfer of proteinaceous material to subsequent instruments from inadequately cleaned brushes.

### Selection of disinfectant

The standard disinfectant for endoscope reprocessing in the UK used to be 2% alkaline-buffered glutaraldehyde. Concerns about the safety of glutaraldehyde have persuaded many departments to try one of the new alternative products aimed at endoscope disinfection. These are generally based on peracetic acid, chlorine dioxide, superoxidized water and or-thophthalaldehyde. As the formulation of products all vary from each other, it is not possible to make the same general recommendations about exposure times as when very similar glutaraldehyde formulations were the accepted standard. The following criteria should be considered for assessment of possible endoscope disinfectants:

**Efficacy.** The agent should have proven efficacy against bacteria (including bacterial spores for invasive endoscopes), mycobacteria and viruses.

**Compatibility** with the endoscopes and processing equipment. An endorsement of compatibility from the endoscope manufacturers should be obtained.

**User safety.** The disinfectant should not cause respiratory or skin problems to the user. Can the product be safely contained to protect the user from any harmful effects? What personal protective equipment is necessary?

**Costs.** The costs of the disinfectant with regard to its use-life, and the costs of any protective ventilation and other equipment should be included.

The properties of a variety of relevant disinfectants may be found in Table 6 and Chapter 2.

It is important to follow the manufacturer's recommendations for effective, safe use at all times and to ensure that all endoscope surfaces are in contact with the disinfectant at an effective concentration for the recommended contact time. If disinfectants are reused, they will become diluted. Test kits/strips should be available for determining the concentration and their use is encouraged. A pattern for renewing the disinfectant should be established by initial extensive observation, with periodic observation thereafter to ensure that parameters have not changed.

## Rinsing

It is important to remove disinfectant residues which may lead to irritation of the patient's mucosa. Heat-sterilized or filtered bacteria-free water is recommended for the final rinse of bronchoscopes, cystoscopes and endoscopes used for endoscopic retrograde cholangiopancreatography (ERCP). In practice, the use of heat-sterilized water is often impractical so filtered bacteria-free water is the most widely used option. The final, bacteria-retentive filters will require protection from blockage with coarser particulate filters preceding them. Current UK recommendations (NHS Estates Agency, 1997) are that this water should be assessed by total

**Table 6:** Properties of instrument disinfectants

| Disinfectant | Microbicidal activity | | | Viruses | | Stable | Inactivation by organic matter | Corrosive/ damaging | Irritant (I) Sensitizing (S) Flammable (F) |
| | Spores | Mycobacteria | Bacteria | Enveloped | Non-enveloped | | | | |
|---|---|---|---|---|---|---|---|---|---|
| Glutaraldehyde | Moderate 3 h | Good 20 min | Good <5 min | Good <5 min | Good <5 min | Moderate (e.g. 14–28 days) | No, but does not penetrate (fixative) | No | I, S |
| Orthophthalaldehyde (0.55%) | Poor > 6 h | Good <5 min | Good <5 min | Good <5 min | Good <5 min | Moderate (30 days) | No but does not penetrate (fixative) | No (staining) | I† |
| Peracetic acid 0.2–0.35%* | Varies 10–20 min | Varies 5–20 min | Good <5 min | Good <5 min | Good <5 min | No (1–3 days) | No | Slight | I |
| Alcohol (usually 70%) | None | Good <5 min | Good <5 min | Good <5 min | Poor to moderate | Yes | No, but does not penetrate (fixative) | Slight (to lens cements) | F |
| Chlorine dioxide | Good <10 min | Good <5 min | Good <5 min | Good <5 min | Good <5 min | No (1–5 days) | Yes | Slight | I |
| Superoxidized water | Good <10 min | Good <5 min | Good <5 min | Good <5 min | Good <5 min | No (<1 day) | Yes | Slight | No |

* Activity varies with concentration of product.
† Anaphylaxis-like reactions have been observed following repeated cystoscopy with instruments disinfected by OPA (Medicines and Healthcare Products Regulatory Agency, 2004).

viable bacterial count on duplicate 100-ml samples on a weekly basis and for mycobacteria on an annual basis.

## Automated endoscope washer-disinfectors

The use of an automated washer-disinfector should be the standard method used for endoscope reprocessing. These should provide a reproducible, standardized method of processing with process controls.

The user should ensure that the washer-disinfector:

- Thoroughly cleans all internal and external surfaces and lumens.
- Disinfects instruments with an effective non-damaging disinfectant at use-concentration and temperature. Single-use disinfectants are preferred as they eliminate the dilution and inactivation effect.
- Removes disinfectant residues with sterile or bacteria-free water.
- Has a self-disinfecting facility, easily operated.
- Contains or removes all chemical vapour emissions.
- Produces a record for cycle validation and instrument/patient traceability.

Systems should be in place to ensure that all channel irrigation occurs, that the disinfectant is above the minimum effective concentration and that the quality of the water is acceptable for the endoscopes being processed.

## Accessories

All accessories should be thoroughly cleaned, preferably using ultrasonics. Many of the reusable accessories associated with endoscopy (e.g. biopsy forceps, injection needles, water bottles etc.) will now withstand autoclaving; consequently a sterile supplies department tray service should be used. Single-use accessories such as biopsy forceps are now preferred by many users and their use should be encouraged if the costs are acceptable.

## Testing and maintenance of endoscope washer-disinfectors

Guidelines on the validation of endoscope washer-disinfectors is given in Health Technical Memorandum 2030 (NHS Estates Agency, 1997). Numerous tests are described for daily, weekly, quarterly and yearly testing. It may not be practical to carry out all of these tests, but as a minimum the user should ensure that all endoscope channels are irrigated, that the disinfectant is above the minimum effective concentration recommended by the manufacturers and that the microbiological quality of the final rinse water is suitable for the endoscopes being processed.

## Babies' incubators

Thorough cleaning with a detergent, paying particular attention to the ports, handles and mattresses, followed by drying is usually adequate. If disinfection is required, the surfaces may be wiped over with a weak solution of a chlorine-based agent (125 ppm av Cl) and a compatible detergent. Wiping with 70% alcohol after cleaning will disinfect, but care is necessary to avoid damage to plastics. Care should be taken to aerate the incubator before reuse. Some humidifiers within the incubator can be disinfected by raising the temperature of the water to over 70°C, or can be removed and autoclaved. Formaldehyde cabinets are also effective, but cleaning is still necessary and care must be taken to aerate to ensure removal of formaldehyde. Formaldehyde disinfectors are expensive and should not be required in most hospitals, but if available should be sited in the hospital's sterile supplies department since careful control is required for efficacy and safety.

## References

British Society of Gastroenterology. (2003) *Guidelines for decontamination of equipment for gastrointestinal endoscopy.* [Available on the British Society of Gastroenterology website at: http://www.bsg.org.uk/pdf_word_docs/disinfection.doc]

British Thoracic Society Bronchoscopy Guidelines Committee, a Subcommittee of Standards of Care Committee of British Thoracic Society. (2001) British Thoracic Society guidelines on diagnostic flexible bronchoscopy. *Thorax* **56** (Suppl 1), 1–21.

Cooke RPD, Feneley RC, Ayliffe G, Lawrence WT, Emmerson AM, Greengrass SM. (1993) Decontamination of Urological Equipment: Interim Report of a Working Group of the Standing Committee on Urological Instruments of the British Association of Urological Surgeons. *British Journal of Urology* **71**, 5–9.

Medical Devices Agency. (2002) *Device Bulletin: Decontamination of Endoscopes* MDA DB(2002)05. Medical Devices Agency, London.

NHS Estates Agency. (1997) *Washer-disinfectors: Validation and verification: Health technical memorandum 2030.* NHS Estates, Leeds. ISBN: 0113220715.

## Further reading

Ayliffe GAJ (Chair of the Minimal Access Therapy Decontamination Working Group). (2000) Decontamination of minimally invasive surgical instruments and accessories. *Journal of Hospital Infection* **45**, 263–277.

Fraise AP, Lambert P, Maillard J-Y, eds. (2003) *Russell, Hugo & Ayliffe's Principles and Practice of Disinfection, Preservation and Sterilization*, 4th edn. Blackwell Science, Oxford. ISBN: 1405101997.

Hospital Infection Society. (2002) Rinse water for heat labile endoscopy equipment. Report from a joint working group of the Hospital Infection Society and the Public Health Laboratory Service. *Journal of Hospital Infection* **51**, 7–16.

Medical Devices Agency Safety Notice. (2002) *Management of loaned medical devices, equipment or accessories from manufacturers or other hospitals.* MDA SN2002(17). Medical Devices Agency, London.

Medicines and Healthcare Products Regulatory Agency. (2003) *Management of medical devices prior to repair, service or investigation.* MHRA DB2003(05). Medicines and Healthcare Products Regulatory Agency, London.

Medicines and Healthcare Products Regulatory Agency. (2004) *Cidex® OPA orthophthalaldehyde high level disinfectant solution.* Medical Device Alert: MDA/2004/022. Medicines and Healthcare Products Regulatory Agency, London.

Microbiology Advisory Committee to the Department of Health. (1996) *Sterilization, Disinfection and Cleaning of Medical Equipment.* Department of Health, London. ISBN: 18858395186. [This document is updated periodically and current versions can be found on the website of the Medicines and Healthcare products Regulatory Agency: http://www.mhra.gov.uk/]

Nelson DB. (2003) Infection control during gastrointestinal infection. *Journal of Laboratory and Clinical Medicine* **141**, 159–167.

NHS Estates Agency. (1997) *Washer-disinfectors: Operational management: Health technical memorandum 2030.* NHS Estates, Leeds. ISBN: 0113220707.

NHS Estates Agency. (1997) *Washer-disinfectors: Design considerations: Health technical memorandum 2030.* NHS Estates, Leeds. ISBN: 0113220693.

# 9 Disinfectants in pathology departments

## The requirements for chemical disinfectants in laboratories

The Approved Codes of Practice to the Control of Substances Hazardous to Health ('COSHH') Regulations (Health and Safety Executive, 2002) require that, with respect to biological agents, laboratories have specified disinfection procedures. Guidance produced by the Advisory Committee on Dangerous Pathogens (2001), a body appointed by the Health and Safety Commission, requires that there are disinfection protocols in place both for routine use and for use in spills, and that workers are trained how to deal with spillages and other forms of contamination. The Health Services Advisory Committee, also appointed by the Health and Safety Commission, has a publication *Safe working and the prevention of infection in clinical laboratories and similar facilities* (2003a) which has an appendix devoted to 'Disinfectants and disinfection in the clinical laboratory'.

## Discard containers

The use of chemical disinfectants is a process of lower quality assurance than other available decontamination procedures such as steam sterilization. Wherever possible, contaminated discarded items should be collected in leakproof vessels, which can then be steam sterilized; incineration is sometimes acceptable as an alternative. A fully loaded discard vessel should periodically be monitored thermometrically to ensure adequate heating in all parts of the load. As well as superior quality assurance of decontamination, use of 'dry discard' removes possible toxic hazards from chemical disinfectants and the need for COSHH risk assessments on the use of those disinfectants (see Chapter 10 for more detailed information on COSHH risk assessments). The practice of putting small volumes of chemical disinfectant into these vessels serves no purpose; most of the contaminated items will be out of contact with the disinfectant, whilst still entailing the disadvantages of chemical disinfectant use just listed.

Where discard pots must still be used, such as for reusable heat-sensitive equipment, hypochlorite or NaDCC at around 2500 ppm av Cl is usually the disinfectant of first choice, with clear soluble phenolics as a possible alternative for bacteriology laboratories. It should be made up freshly at the start of each working day and left overnight before discarding the following morning. Hypochlorites are prone to inactivation by organic matter (though 2500 ppm av Cl should be able to withstand a considerable amount) and can, from time to time, be checked for inactivation before disposal. Starch–iodide paper, which will show the presence of strong oxidizing agents, will turn a blue-black colour in the presence of hypochlorite and hypochlorous acid (the active components within chlorine-based disinfectants). However, high concentrations of hypochlorite can bleach this colour rapidly. If the paper appears not to change on contact with a hypochlorite solution, dilute a small volume of the test solution about 100-fold. If there was a high hypochlorite concentration in the original, this dilution will turn the paper blue-black. If there was no hypochlorite in the original, it will remain white. If inactivation of the disinfectant is occurring, either less organic matter should be put in the discard pot or a higher concentration of hypochlorite should be used. Clear soluble phenolics should be the first choice where there is a risk of mycobacteria.

Items placed in discard jars must be completely submerged. The disinfectant must be in contact with all the inner surfaces of the items and with their contents. Items must remain in the disinfectant for at least 1 hour and preferably overnight before disposal. The disinfectant must then be emptied down a sink (not a handwash basin) through a sieve or colander. Reusable items may be washed and reprocessed after overnight submersion.

## Spills

There is a requirement (Advisory Committee on Dangerous Pathogens, 2001) to have adequate plans for dealing with accidents, the majority of which are likely to be spills. The assessment of risk from a spill and how to negate that risk is a much wider topic than just the choice of a disinfectant to use on that spill. It will involve, amongst other things, judgement of an individual's exposure and how to minimize hazards from that. Spills should be cleared either by covering with a liquid disinfectant or with absorbent disinfectant granules, left for a few minutes and then carefully cleared and disposed of as contaminated waste. A chlorine-based agent (e.g. sodium hypochlorite or NaDCC) is usually first choice for use on spills. Single-use gloves should be worn when dealing with a spill. If there is any risk that sharp items, such as broken glass, may be in the spill, scoops or an autoclavable dustpan and brush should be used to clear the disinfected spill. Eye or face protection should be worn. Kits consisting of protective clothing, disinfectant, scoop etc. are commercially available.

Small spills can be cleared by wiping the contaminated surface with a suitable disinfectant, but a wide area around the visible spill should also be treated; small splashes generated from the original spill may not be visible.

## Room fumigation

Large spills of high-risk material in a containment level 3 laboratory may disperse to such an extent that decontamination by local application of liquid chemical is an unreliable option (Tearle, 2003). All UK containment level 3 laboratories must be sealable to permit disinfection (Health and Safety Executive, 2002); such disinfection is best effected by formaldehyde fumigation. In practice, this means that the room should be sealed except for the door, which can be sealed with tape, and any air transfer grille in the door, which can be sealed with plastic sheeting and tape, after the fumigation has been set up. It will require regular, at least annual, reassessments to ensure that a room remains sealable. Room fumigation is a very hazardous procedure. If a room under fumigation leaks, there is a severe hazard to people in surrounding areas and, if sufficient formaldehyde vapour is lost, there may be inadequate decontamination inside the room. Commercial formalin is a stabilized solution containing 40% formaldehyde. A formula found to be effective is to boil off a mixture of 100 ml formalin and 900 ml water for every 28.3 $m^3$ (1000 $ft^3$) room space (Jones, 1995). Fumigation should be for at least 6 hours, and preferably overnight. The room should be capable of being vented safely without the need to enter it. Even if this is the case, at least two people equipped with self-contained breathing apparatus and trained in its use should be present in case of untoward occurrence, such as the room leaking and the fumigation having to be terminated rapidly. Gas samples for formaldehyde levels should be taken through a small, sealable hole in the door. The room can be entered when the level is below 2 ppm, but polymerized formaldehyde deposited on surfaces can continue to generate formaldehyde vapour for a considerable time following fumigation. Fumigation may not penetrate central areas of spills if they contain high levels of organic matter or are occluded by debris or other matter. These should be treated with an appropriate disinfectant after fumigation has decontaminated dispersed splashes and aerosols and made the room safe to enter.

## Safety cabinet fumigation

Small spills in a safety cabinet can be treated by local disinfection, as for 'Spills' above. Larger spills within a microbiological safety cabinet should be well contained, but splashes might have contaminated the worker's gloved hands and lab coat; these should be changed. Safety cabinets are readily decontaminated by fumigation. A volume of 25 ml formalin should be generated inside a sealed standard-sized cabinet using an electric heater. The practice of boiling off formaldehyde by adding 10 g potassium permanganate to 35 ml formalin is not recommended; the mixture boils rapidly and can be hazardous to a worker who does not manage to seal the safety cabinet before this happens. As with rooms, fumigation should be for at least 6 hours, preferably overnight. It must be ensured that there is no-one in the vicinity of the safety cabinet outlet when it is vented after fumigation. Safety cabinet fumigation is recommended after a spill and prior to service or repair of the cabinet.

## Decontamination of equipment before service or repair

If equipment may have become contaminated during use, it must be decontaminated before it is serviced or repaired, either *in situ* or at a remote location (Medicines and Healthcare Products Regulatory Agency, 2003). A decontamination certificate should be completed for each occasion and should state either that the item was not initially contaminated, that it has been successfully decontaminated, or that it cannot be decontaminated, and advice should be given on the nature of any hazard and measures necessary to work on the equipment safely.

An alcohol wipe applied to a physically clean surface and which remains wet with disinfectant for at least 1 minute, can be used to disinfect the surfaces of equipment (e.g. electrical equipment) for which immersion or soaking in disinfectant is impractical. (Remember that alcohols are flammable. Care must be taken where equipment may generate heat or sparks.) A wipe with a clear soluble phenolic can be used if the contamination is with vegetative bacteria or enveloped viruses.

## Centrifuges

Loads should be sealed during centrifugation; if they are, the routine disinfection of centrifuges is not necessary. If a load is not sealed and causes contamination, then periodic disinfection will not negate any risk; the centrifuge should be modified or replaced. Disinfection may be necessary before a centrifuge is serviced or repaired, or when it is suspected that tubes may have broken or leaked during centrifugation. Following an actual or suspected breakage or leak, the lid should be kept closed (or rapidly reclosed on discovery of the breakage) for at least 30 minutes to allow aerosols to settle. Protective gloves must be worn, and forceps or swabs held in forceps used to pick up glass debris. Broken glass, buckets, trunnions and the rotor must be autoclaved or placed in a non-corrosive disinfectant (i.e. not hypochlorite) known to be effective against the organisms concerned and approved by the centrifuge manufacturer as compatible with the centrifuge, and left for at least 10–20 minutes. Unbroken, capped tubes may be placed in the disinfectant in a separate container for at least 10–20 minutes and the contents then recovered. The centrifuge bowl must be swabbed with disinfectant, left to dry, then swabbed again, and finally wiped with water and dried.

## Automated equipment used in chemical pathology laboratories

Automated equipment should not disperse contamination. If it does, it should be modified or replaced; periodic disinfection will not negate any risk. Surfaces that may become contaminated should be disinfected periodically, at least at the end of each day. The equipment may need disinfection before maintenance or repair. In normal circumstances it is only necessary to decontaminate the liquid lines of automated equipment that are in direct contact with samples and any outer surfaces of such equipment that has contact with contamination. After washing through with water the liquid lines can be flushed with strong solution of a chlorine-based agent (2500 ppm av Cl), provided that no metal components are involved, or another disinfectant with a suitable microbicidal range that is approved by the equipment manufacturer. If contamination of the outside of the machine is known or suspected, the surfaces should be cleaned, dried and wiped with an alcohol solution.

## Work benches

If a spill is known or suspected, work benches should be decontaminated as for 'Spills' above. Even if no contamination is suspected, small, inapparent splashes are likely to have occurred and they should be wiped with a suitable disinfectant periodically and at the end of each working day (Advisory Committee on Dangerous Pathogens, 2001). A chlorine-based agent at 1000–2500 ppm av Cl can be used, or 70% alcohol if the surface is physically clean and there is no fire risk from using an inflammable, volatile liquid.

## Hands

Hand contamination acquired whilst working in a clinical laboratory will be located superficially on the skin and will be readily removed. Washing with plain soap or detergent should be sufficient. Any handwashing agent must be capable of being used many times a day without causing skin problems. Surgical scrubs are unlikely to add significantly to decontamination (they are primarily designed to suppress regrowth of the microflora resident on the skin) and can cause drying and cracking of skin if used frequently. A rapid alternative to washing is the use of an alcohol handrub. If a small volume (2–3 ml) of around 70% either ethanol (usually as industrial methylated spirit) or isopropanol is rubbed to dryness on the hands, it produces decontamination equivalent to washing. Such handrubs can be obtained commercially as gels or liquids.

Gloves frequently develop holes during use. Liquid contamination on the outside of a hole will wick through to the inside by capillary action. Hands should always be washed immediately after gloves are removed.

## Use of disinfectants in the mortuary and post-mortem room

Contaminated surfaces need to be cleaned and, if a case may be high risk, disinfected between cases, and cleaned and disinfected at the end of each day. The most common environmental disinfectants in use in mortuaries and post-mortem rooms are clear soluble phenolics and hypochlorites (Health Services Advisory Committee, 2003b), but others can be considered as appropriate for local circumstances. Care must be taken not to let hypochlorites mix with formaldehyde: bis (chloromethyl) ether, a carcinogen, may be formed (Gamble, 1977).

The first choice for instrument decontamination should be thermal, either disinfection in a thermal washer-disinfector or cleaning followed by steam sterilization. Use of a washer-disinfector removes much of the risk from handling instruments during the manual cleaning prior to steam sterilization. Small bench-top washer-disinfectors are now available. Washer-disinfectors used in post-mortem rooms may not require the same level of testing as those used for surgical instruments.

Instruments can be disinfected by cleaning, followed by immersion in a chemical disinfectant that has a suitable microbicidal range and will not corrode the instrument. This lacks the high quality assurance of thermal processes but may be more appropriate for some complex or heat-intolerant instruments.

For cadavers which are definitely, probably, suspected or at risk of CJD, single-use instruments should be used wherever possible and disposed of by incineration. Where this is not feasible, a dedicated instrument set should be used for such cases (Advisory Committee on Dangerous Pathogens and Spongiform Encephalopathy Advisory Committee, 2003). Dispersion of contaminated material should be minimized. Working surfaces should be decontaminated by repeated wetting for 1 hour with 20 000 ppm av Cl from sodium hydroxide or 2 M sodium hydroxide.

## References

Advisory Committee on Dangerous Pathogens. (2001) *The Management, Design and Operation of Microbiological Containment Laboratories.* HSE Books, Sudbury. ISBN: 0717620344.

Advisory Committee on Dangerous Pathogens and Spongiform Encephalopathy Advisory Committee. (2003) *Transmissible spongiform encephalopathy agents: safe working and the prevention of infection.* Published on the UK Department of Health website at: http://www.dh.gov.uk.

Gamble MR. (1977) Hazard: formaldehyde and hypochlorites. *Laboratory Animals* **11**, 61.

Health and Safety Executive. (2002) *Control of Substances Hazardous to Health Regulations, 2002,* 4th edn. HSE Books, Sudbury. ISBN: 0717625346.

Health Services Advisory Committee. (2003a) *Safe working and prevention of infection in clinical laboratories and similar facilities.* HSE Books, Sudbury. ISBN: 0717625133.

Health Services Advisory Committee. (2003b) *Safe working and prevention of infection in the mortuary and post-mortem rooms.* HSE Books, Sudbury. ISBN: 0717622932.

Jones BPC. (1995) Fumigation and the management of containment level 3 facilities. *PHLS Microbiology Digest* **12**, 169–171.

Medicines and Healthcare Products Regulatory Agency. (2003) *Device Bulletin 2003(05). Management of Medical Devices Prior to Repair, Service or Investigation.* Medicines and Healthcare Products Regulatory Agency, London.

Tearle P. (2003) Decontamination by fumigation. *Communicable Disease and Public Health* **6**, 166–168.

## Further reading

Collins CH, Kennedy DA. (1999) *Laboratory-Acquired Infections: History, Incidence, Causes and Prevention,* 4th edn. Butterworth Heinmann, Oxford. ISBN: 0750640235.

# 10 Safety in chemical disinfection

There is an increasing emphasis on safety in all aspects of work practice. Many chemical disinfectants can cause harmful effects in those who use them. This section reflects the approach to safety aspects of the use of chemical disinfectants at the time of writing in the UK. Specific legal issues will vary between countries and with time.

## Control of Substances Hazardous to Health Regulations

In the UK, the main legal control over the use of chemical disinfectants is covered by the Control of Substances Hazardous to Health Regulations (2002): 'COSHH'. These require employers to control exposures to hazardous substances to protect both employees and any others who may be exposed from work activities. Hazardous substances within COSHH are anything that can harm the health of people who work with them if the substances are not properly controlled.

Under COSHH, employers must:

- assess the risks to health arising from the work;
- decide what precautions are needed;
- prevent or control people's exposure;
- ensure that the control measures are used and maintained;
- if necessary, monitor exposure and carry out health surveillance;
- ensure employees are properly informed, trained and supervised.

All possibly harmful substances should have a safety data sheet, written by the suppliers, giving relevant information about the products. These, and any other sources of information, should be used to prepare a risk assessment on their use and, if appropriate, their storage and disposal. This risk assessment, a record of which should be kept, is an evaluation of the substance, the risks it presents and the precautions that might need to be taken under the actual conditions of use. It should enable an employer to make valid decisions about controlling health risks from hazardous substances and to show how these decisions were arrived at. If a risk assessment shows that there are no health risks or that the risk is trivial, no more action is needed. If there are health risks, then employers must consider what else needs to be done to comply fully with COSHH requirements.

This process should:

- Work out what hazardous substances are used in the workplace and find out the risks from using these substances to people's health.
- Establish if a safer alternative is available.
- Decide what precautions are needed before working with these substances. Ideally, these precautions should prevent people being exposed to the hazardous substances, but where this is not reasonably practicable, any exposure should be controlled.
- Ensure that the control measures are used and maintained properly and that safety procedures are followed.
- If required, monitor exposure of employees to the hazardous substances.
- Carry out health surveillance where an assessment has shown that this is necessary, or if COSHH makes this a specific requirement.
- If required, prepare plans and procedures to deal with accidents, incidents and emergencies.
- Ensure that employees are properly informed, trained and supervised.

Microbial pathogens are also covered by COSHH if they are directly connected to the work, such as in laboratories, or if exposure is incidental to work, such as in healthcare. Thus chemical disinfectants in healthcare can be both a problem and a solution under COSHH.

The general philosophy of the COSHH regulations is that procedures, rather than substances, should be assessed for risk. This takes into account the substance, the nature of its use, the likely exposure of people to the substance and measures taken to limit that exposure. Thus the use of, for example, an alcohol skin wipe would not pose the same risk as a chemical tanker transporting several thousand litres of alcohol. The emphasis of the regulations is on prevention of exposure to hazardous substances. Personal protective equipment such as gloves, respiratory and eye protection, aprons etc. should only be used to prevent exposure as a last resort or in addition to other methods.

Exposure to chemical disinfectants can be through direct contact with skin or mucous membranes or by inhalation. The inhalation exposure limit to a chemical is expressed as an occupational exposure limit (OEL). OELs are expressed as the chemical concentration in the working atmosphere and are published periodically by the UK Health and Safety Executive in a document in the 'EH40' series (HSE, 2003). OELs can be expressed in two ways: a maximum exposure limit (MEL); and an occupational exposure standard (OES). An MEL is for limited-term exposure, either short term, a reference period of 15 minutes, or long term, a time-weighted average over 8 hours. Short-term exposure limits are set to help prevent effects such as eye irritation, which may occur following exposure for a few minutes. MELs are set for substances which may cause the most serious health effects, such as cancer and occupational asthma. COSHH requires that exposure should be reduced as far below the MEL as is reasonably practicable and, if the chemical has a short-term (15-minute) MEL, exposure must never exceed the MEL during the reference period. An OES relates to longer-term exposure and is set at a level at which, based on current knowledge of an average 8-hour exposure, there is no indication of risk to the health of workers who breathe it in day after day. If exposure to a substance that has an OES is reduced at least to that level, then adequate control has been achieved. Precise instructions on how to apply MELs and OESs can be found in EH40 (Health and Safety Executive, 2001) which interprets Regulation 7 of COSHH (Health and Safety Executive, 2002). If a substance has neither an MEL nor an OES, this does not necessarily mean it is safe. It should still be controlled to levels which are as low as reasonably practicable and which, day after day, have no effects on health. Information on exposure levels should be available from suppliers, manufacturers and trade associations.

The possible hazards of exposure via skin must also be taken into account. This can result from direct splashing to skin or to clothing or, in exceptional circumstances, from a high atmospheric concentration of a chemical. Absorption through skin can result in very high exposure levels.

## Possible changes in COSHH

The Health and Safety Commission is currently re-evaluating exposure to chemicals at work. It is currently proposed that the existing system of OEL and MEL be replaced by a system based on workplace exposure limits (WELs). A WEL will be a value that should not be exceeded; in effect similar to an MEL, but which can apply to all, not just the more toxic, chemicals listed. There will also be an increased emphasis on the role of good practice in controlling exposure to substances hazardous to health.

## COSHH and chemical disinfectants

The risk from chemicals must be assessed with reference to the toxic properties of that chemical, the amount handled and the manner of its use.

A chemical that may be extremely hazardous in its concentrated form, chlorine for example, is beneficial and safe when used in a diluted, controlled manner as a swimming pool disinfectant, producing minor irritation at most. Thus chemical disinfectants can present two levels of risk. The greater risk is from undiluted disinfectants and should be assessed separately from the diluted preparations. Concentrated disinfectants should always be stored and handled with care. The original container should be the safest storage vessel, designed to minimize any risks that the disinfectant may pose such as flammability or pressure build-up. It should also have clear labelling as to the nature of any hazards. Both these advantages could be lost if the disinfectant is decanted or repackaged in inappropriate vessels.

In preparing a risk assessment, replacing a hazardous agent with a less hazardous one, or an alternative procedure such as thermal decontamination processes, should always be one of the prime considerations. If this is not possible, total or partial enclosure of the chemical, with suitable local exhaust ventilation, must be considered. Prevention of skin contamination is also important. The less manipulation of concentrated solutions there is, the lower the risk of uncontrolled exposure. Splashes and spills occur mostly when concentrated solutions are poured out. The less this happens, the fewer accidents will occur. Such dilution should, where feasible, be done in a controlled, well-equipped environment, such as a pharmacy, rather than on a ward. If dilution on a ward is preferred, use of a solid, tabletted form of disinfectant may present less hazard than concentrated liquid disinfectants. Where necessary, personal protective equipment should be used when manipulating concentrated disinfectants. This should be chosen with regard to the areas of the operator's body that are at risk of exposure, their susceptibility to the agent and consideration of the nature of the hazard. Thus, where the risk is of vapour inhalation, surgical or particulate filter masks play no protective role as they provide no barrier to vapour-phase. Similarly, gloves should be chosen with consideration of their chemical resistances and permeabilities.

Safety data sheets are available from disinfectant manufacturers and will provide additional data to help formulate risk assessments for use of a product.

## Individual disinfectants: safety notes

Occupational exposure standards can be obtained from a current version of the publication EH40, published by the Health and Safety Executive and periodically updated. The figures quoted are from EH40/2002, taking into account an addendum published in 2003 (HSE, 2003). Safety data in other contexts can be obtained from safety data sheets supplied by the manufacturer or supplier or from chemical safety databases, such as that of the International Labour Organization.

## Chlorine

OES: 1 ppm or 2.9 mg m$^{-3}$ for a 15-minute reference period and 0.5 ppm or 1.5 mg m$^{-3}$ for 8-hour time-weighted average reference period.

## Chlorine dioxide

OES: 0.3 ppm or 0.84 mg m$^{-3}$ for a 15-minute reference period and 0.1 ppm or 0.28 mg m$^{-3}$ for 8-hour time-weighted average reference period.

## Ethanol (usually as industrial methylated spirit)

OES: 1000 ppm or 1920 mg m$^{-3}$ for 8-hour time-weighted average reference period. Flammable.

## Formaldehyde

MEL: 2 ppm or 2.5 mg m$^{-3}$ for both 15-minute reference period and 8-hour time-weighted average reference period. Potent eye and nasal irritant. Can cause respiratory distress and allergic dermatitis. Formaldehyde should not be used in the presence of hypochlorites. They may react to form bis (chloromethyl) ether, a carcinogen (Gamble, 1977).

## Glutaraldehyde

MEL: 0.05 ppm or 0.2 mg m$^{-3}$ for both 15-minute reference period and 8-hour time-weighted average reference period. Glutaraldehyde is a respiratory sensitizer.

The use of glutaraldehyde is becoming increasingly problematic, purely for health and safety reasons. It is an eye and nasal irritant, as well as being listed as an respiratory sensitizer ('asthmagen') by the UK Health and Safety Executive. Such agents can produce asthma in individuals exposed in the workplace, or can irritate the respiratory tract in individuals with pre-existing asthma. Once sensitized, individuals can experience respiratory symptoms at below the exposure limits.

## Hydrogen peroxide

OES: 2 ppm or 2.8 mg m$^{-3}$ for a 15-minute reference period and 1 ppm or 1.4 mg m$^{-3}$ for 8-hour time-weighted average reference period.

Strong solutions may be irritant to the skin and mucous membranes. High pressure can develop in sealed containers.

## Hypochlorites

Safety precautions should be based on the manufacturer's or supplier's safety data sheet. Concentrated solutions can cause burns or irritation to skin.

Hypochlorites can release gaseous chlorine if acidified. NaDCC is more prone than alkaline sodium hypochlorite preparations to giving off chlorine, for example when being used to disinfect some large urine spills that may be slightly acidic. Hypochlorites should not be used in the presence of formaldehyde. They may react to form bis (chloromethyl) ether, a carcinogen (Gamble, 1977).

## Iodine

OES: 0.1 ppm or 1.1 mg m$^{-3}$ for a 15-minute reference period. Iodine as alcoholic solution ('tincture') and as a solution in potassium iodine ('Lugol's') can cause skin and eye irritation. Iodine as an alcoholic solution is flammable.

## Orthophthalaldehyde (OPA)

A high molecular weight dialdehyde. Safety precautions should be based on the manufacturer's or supplier's safety data sheet.

## Peracetic acid

Peracetic acid does not have an OES and is currently under review by the Health and Safety Executive. Safety precautions should be based on the manufacturer's or supplier's safety data sheet. Exists as an equilibrium with hydrogen peroxide and acetic acid. The presence of these chemicals should also be taken into account.

## Phenolic disinfectants (clear soluble phenolics, white fluids, black fluids)

These are complex mixtures of phenol-based molecules, the nature and proportion of which will vary between products. Safety precautions should be based on the manufacturer's or supplier's safety data sheet.

## Phenol

MEL: 2 ppm 8-hour time-weighted average reference period. Can be absorbed through skin.

## Propan-1-ol (propanol)

OES: 250 ppm or 625 mg m$^{-3}$ for a 15-minute reference period and 200 ppm or 500 mg m$^{-3}$ for 8-hour time-weighted average reference period. Flammable. Can be absorbed through skin.

## Propan-2-ol (isopropanol)

OES: 500 ppm or 1250 mg m$^{-3}$ for a 15-minute reference period and 400 ppm or 999 mg m$^{-3}$ for 8-hour time-weighted average reference period. Flammable.

## References

Gamble MR. (1977) Hazard: formaldehyde and hypochlorite. *Laboratory Animals* **11**, 61.

Health and Safety Executive. (2002) *Control of Substances Hazardous to Health,* 4th edn. *Approved Code of Practice and Guidance.* HSE Books, London. ISBN: 0717625346

Health and Safety Executive. (2001) *EH40/02: Occupational Exposure Limits 2002.* HSE Books, London. ISBN 0717620832, with ammendments in the 2003 supplement, ISBN 0717621723.

## Further reading

Collins CH, Kennedy DA. (1999) *Laboratory-Acquired Infections: History, Incidence, Causes and Prevention,* 4th edn. Butterworth Heinmann, Oxford. ISBN: 0750640235.

# 11 Disinfectant testing

Ideally, disinfectant testing should inform users about how a disinfectant will perform in a given situation and allow them to compare the attributes of different products. The more a test replicates the conditions under which a disinfectant is used, the more that test will predict its performance in use. However, to be reproducible, disinfectant tests need to be highly controlled. This contrasts with the majority of actual disinfectant use, where conditions can be highly variable. So at best, the testing of disinfectants can be a broad guide to their efficacy in actual use but cannot guarantee that they will achieve acceptable disinfection in a given situation. The conditions of use and properties of the disinfectant also need to be taken into consideration.

Testing disinfectants goes back to near the origins of microbiology in the 1880s when Robert Koch inoculated anthrax spores onto silk threads, immersed these in disinfectants and then cultured the threads in growth media or test animals. One of the first standardized assessments of disinfectant activity was the Rideal–Walker test (Rideal & Walker, 1903), which compared a test disinfectant with a standard disinfectant (phenol), the result being expressed as a ratio of activities: a 'phenol coefficient'. This was modified to include organic matter (initially dried faeces, later replaced by yeast) in the Chick–Martin test; again a phenol coefficient test. The concept of comparing a disinfectant to an arbitrary reference compound generates limited information on the attributes of a disinfectant and how to use it. Despite this, phenol coefficients were internationally common until the 1960s. Meanwhile there was parallel development of tests that reproduced the actual conditions in which disinfectants were used. Disinfectant inactivators also started to be used, preventing an apparent enhancement of microbicidal activity caused by disinfectant carry-over into the recovery phase. In the UK, the Kelsey–Sykes test, first published in 1969, with an improved version in 1974 (Kelsey & Maurer, 1974), modelled the progressive dilution and pollution that a disinfectant may get during use and included neutralization of the disinfectant on sampling. The result given by this test was a disinfectant concentration appropriate for use in either clean or dirty conditions, rather than an arbitrary comparison.

The multiplicity of chemical disinfectant tests of the various European national standardization bodies are at present being replaced by a series of tests formulated by the European Committee for Standardization (CEN). These standards have three sequential phases: In phase 1 tests, the basic microbicidal ability of a preparation is ascertained. Phase 2 tests simulate use conditions: phase 2, step 1 tests are suspension tests and phase 2, step 2 tests are surface tests, which include skin disinfection. Phase 3 tests will eventually be field trials of a disinfectant (none are currently formulated). There will be specific tests for disinfectants with medical applications, as well as other fields such as veterinary, food, industrial and domestic areas. The CEN disinfectant tests are based on the rate of kill; they require a specified minimum reduction of the test microbial levels in a specified time. The reduction is usually $10^5$ (i.e. a 100 000-fold) and the time of exposure can vary, typically between 1 and 60 minutes, according to the exposure likely to occur in practice. The tests require the use of neutralizers to ensure that the residual activity of disinfectant carried-over during sampling does not affect results; neutralizers have to be validated for each disinfectant tested. An organic load is used to simulate realistic use conditions in phase 2, step 1 tests.

The groups of organisms used as targets in these tests are bacteria, (including mycobacteria, *Legionella pneumophila* and bacterial spores), viruses (including bacteriophage) or fungi (including yeasts). Generally, each test nominates specific strains of test species, with additional strains that can be used when appropriate. When the target is the resident skin microflora, the bacteria already present on volunteers' skin are used. When the target is transient skin contaminants, micro-organisms are applied to skin.

## Outlines of current CEN tests relevant to medical applications

### Phase 1 tests

There is one basic test for bactericidal and one for fungicidal activity. The basic test for bactericidal activity EN 1040 (British Standards Institution, 1997a) determines that at least a 100 000-fold (5 $\log_{10}$) reduction of *Pseudomonas aeruginosa* and *Staphylococcus aureus* shall be achieved by the use dilution of the disinfectant within 60 minutes. Similarly, a disinfectant tested by the basic fungicidal test EN 1275 (British Standards Institution, 1997b) should show at least a 10 000-fold (4 $\log_{10}$) reduction in *Aspergillus niger* and *Candida albicans* within 60 minutes. These tests are just to indicate whether there is a basic level of bactericidal or fungicidal activity. Suitability for application in a particular intended use should be determined by further tests in the phase 2 series.

## Phase 2 tests

Two phase 2, step 1 suspension tests for medical instrument disinfectants have been published at the time of writing: EN 13727 (British Standards Institution, 2003a) is to determine bactericidal activity and EN 13624 (British Standards Institution, 2003b) is to determine fungicidal activity.

In the test for bactericidal activity, the obligatory test organisms are *Pseudomonas aeruginosa*, *Staphylococcus aureus* and *Enterococcus hirae*. In the test for fungal activity the obligatory test organism is the yeast *Candida albicans*; spores of filamentous fungus *Aspergillus niger* can be used in addition. Both tests use a disinfection time of 60 minutes at 20°C and simulate disinfection in 'clean' and 'dirty' conditions, using albumin and erythrocytes as organic soil. Validated neutralizers must be used in the recovery phase. A bactericidal disinfectant must produce a 5 decimal log (100 000-fold) reduction in all test suspensions; a fungicidal disinfectant must produce a 4 decimal log (10 000-fold) reduction. (If a product passes the test against *C. albicans* only, 'yeasticidal' activity can be claimed; if it passes against *C. albicans* and *Asp. niger*, 'fungicidal' activity can be claimed.)

There are two phase 2, step 2 tests published for handwashing agents. These are EN 1499 (British Standards Institution, 1997c) a test for 'hygienic handwash' formulations and EN 1500 (British Standards Institution, 1997d), a test for 'hygienic handrub' formulations. Both tests involve assessing the removal or destruction of artificially applied transient contamination, *Escherichia coli*, from the hands of 12–15 volunteers. The test products are statistically compared with reference products. EN 1499 uses an unmedicated liquid soap as the reference product and the mean reduction of test bacteria has to be significantly larger than that achieved using the reference product. EN 1500 uses 60% propan-2-ol as the reference product and the mean reduction of test bacteria should not be significantly smaller than that achieved using the reference product.

## Other tests

The phase 2 step 1 tests for the mycobactericidal and virucidal activity of disinfectants are still under formulation. Examples of existing suspension and surface tests for viruses have been described by Sattar *et al.* (1989) and Tyler *et al.* (1990) and for mycobacteria by Griffiths *et al.* (1998) and Best *et al.* (1988). A comprehensive review of test methods can be found in Ayliffe (1989), Block (2001) and Reybrouck (2003).

## In-use disinfectant tests

The efficacy of disinfectants in use can be tested by sampling them for the presence of viable bacteria. Examples of such testing are given by Maurer (1985) and Prince & Ayliffe (1972). In essence, a sample of a disinfectant is taken, neutralized and cultured to enumerate surviving bacteria. The disinfectant and neutralizer can be mixed together, or the disinfectant can be put through a filter, followed by the neutralizer and then the filter placed on a solid growth medium and cultured for survivors. The disinfectant should always be given sufficient time to act before a sample is taken or a positive result will not necessarily indicate disinfectant failure in practice.

Hypochlorites can also be tested in-use with starch–iodide indicator paper. Details are in Chapter 9.

## References

Ayliffe GAJ. (1989) Standardisation of disinfectant testing. *Journal of Hospital Infection* **13**, 211–216.

Best M, Sattar SA, Springthorpe VS & Kennedy ME. (1988) Comparative mycobactericidal activity of chemical disinfectants in suspension and carrier tests. *Applied and Environmental Microbiology* **54**, 2856–2858.

Block SS (ed). (2001) *Disinfection, Sterilization and Preservation*. 5th edn. Lippincott Williams & Wilkins, Philadelphia. ISBN: 0683307401

British Standards Institution. (1997a) EN 1040:1997 *Chemical disinfectants and antiseptics. Basic bactericidal activity. Test method and requirements (phase 1)*. British Standards Institution, London.

British Standards Institution. (1997b) EN 1275:1997 *Chemical disinfectants and antiseptics. Basic fungicidal activity. Test method and requirements (phase 1)*. British Standards Institution, London.

British Standards Institution. (1997c) EN 1499:1997 *Chemical disinfectants and antiseptics. Hygienic handwash. Test method and requirements (phase 2/step 2)*. British Standards Institution, London.

British Standards Institution. (1997d) EN 1500:1997 *Chemical disinfectants and antiseptics. Hygienic handrub. Test method and requirements (phase 2/step 2)*. British Standards Institution, London.

British Standards Institution. (2003a) EN 13727:2003 *Chemical disinfectants and antiseptics. Quantitative suspension test for the evaluation of bactericidal activity of chemical disinfectants for instruments used in the medical area. Test method and requirements (phase 2, step 1)*. British Standards Institution, London.

British Standards Institution. (2003b) EN 13624:2003 *Chemical disinfectants and antiseptics. Quantitative suspension test for the evaluation of fungicidal activity of chemical disinfectants for instruments used in the medical area. Test method and requirements (phase 2, step 1).* British Standards Institution, London.

Griffiths PA, Babb JR, Fraise AP. (1998) *Mycobacterium terrae*: a potential surrogate for Mycobacterium tuberculosis in a standard disinfectant test. *Journal of Hospital Infection* **38**, 183–192.

Kelsey JC, Maurer IM. (1974) An improved (1974) Kelsey-Sykes test for disinfectants. *The Pharmaceutical Journal* **207**, 528-530.

Maurer IM. (1985) *Hospital Hygiene* 3rd edn. Arnold, London. ISBN 0713144432

Prince J, Ayliffe GA. (1972) In-use testing of disinfectants in hospitals. *Journal of Clinical Pathology* **25**, 586–9.

Reybrouck G. (2003) Evaluation of the antibacterial and antifungal activity of disinfectants. In: Fraise AP, Lambert P, Maillard J-Y (eds). *Russell, Hugo & Ayliffe's Principles and Practice of Disinfection, Preservation and Sterilization* 4th edn. Blackwell Science, Oxford. ISBN: 1405101997

Rideal S, Walker JTA. (1903) Standardisation of disinfectants. *Journal of the Sanitary Institute, London* **24**, 424–441.

Sattar SA, Springthorpe VS, Karim Y, Loro P. (1989). Chemical disinfection of non-porous inanimate surfaces with four human pathogenic viruses. *Epidemiology and Infection* **102**, 493–505.

Tyler R, Ayliffe GAJ, Bradley CR. (1990) Virucidal activity of disinfectants: studies with the poliovirus. *Journal of Hospital Infection* **15**, 339–345.

# Appendix: Summary of policy for decontamination of equipment or environment

This summary is modified by kind permission of the publishers from Ayliffe GAJ, Fraise AP, Geddes AM, Mitchell KM, eds. (2000) *Control of Hospital Infection: A practical handbook*, 4th edn. Arnold, London.

Throughout the following policy, the abbreviations listed below have been used to refer to certain categories of disinfection.

Although chlorine-based agents are commonly recommended instead of phenolics for routine disinfection, their use should be avoided where damage to materials (bleaching of fabrics, corrosion of metals) is likely.

Heat    Sterilization is achieved with a steam sterilizer (autoclave) or hot air oven. Thermal disinfection is achieved with a washer-disinfector.

Cl    Chlorine-based agents (see Table 2 for concentrations).

Phen    Clear, soluble phenolics at the use-dilution recommended for 'clean' conditions, unless significant organic matter is present.

Alc    70–90% ethanol or industrial methylated spirit; 60–70% isopropanol. Immersion provides better disinfection than a wipe.

| Equipment | Routine or preferred method | Acceptable alternative or additional recommendations |
|---|---|---|
| Airways and endotracheal tubes and laryngeal mask airways | Single-use or heat disinfection/sterilization | |
| Baths/showers/shower chairs | Non-infected patients: clean with non-abrasive cleaner | Infected patients and before/after patients with open wounds: Cl in compatible formulation |
| Bed-frames | Wash with detergent | In high-risk area or after infected patient, Cl or Phen |
| Bedpans | Heat in washer-disinfector or use single-use and macerator | Wash carriers for single-use pans after use |

*continued p. 94*

| Equipment | Routine or preferred method | Acceptable alternative or additional recommendations |
|---|---|---|
| Bowls (surgical) | Autoclave or single-use | |
| Bowls (patient washing) | Wash and dry, store inverted | For infected patients or in high-risk areas, use individual bowls and disinfect by heat, Cl or Phen on discharge |
| Carpets | Vacuum clean daily (high-efficiency filter on exhaust); clean periodically by hot water extraction | For known contaminated spillage clean with detergent; disinfect with agent which does not damage carpet |
| Crockery and cutlery | Machine wash or hand wash by approved method | For patients with enteric infections or open pulmonary tuberculosis, if possible heat disinfect—if not, use single-use |
| Curtains (bed) | Machine wash with thermal disinfection when soiled or at least twice yearly | With infected patient or in high-risk area, machine wash with thermal disinfection on patient discharge |
| Drains | Do not need disinfection | If drains smell, clean them or seek input from Estates Department |
| Duvets | Water-impermeable cover: wash, cover with detergent solution and dry | If contaminated, heat disinfect cover and duvet if tolerant or chemical disinfect if effective compatible agent available |
| Endoscopes | Heat-tolerant endoscopes: heat sterilize or disinfect. Heat sensitive endoscopes: chemical disinfection with compatible agent | See Chapter 8 |
| Feeding bottles and teats | Presterilized or heat-disinfected feeds | Teats and bottles presterilized. Cl should only be used in small units where other methods are not available |
| Floors (dry cleaning) | Vacuum clean (with high-efficiency filter on exhaust) or dust-attracting dry mop | Do not use brooms in patient areas |
| Floors (wet cleaning) | Wash with detergent solution; disinfection not routinely required | Known contaminated spillage and terminal disinfection: disinfect with compatible agent |

*continued*

| Equipment | Routine or preferred method | Acceptable alternative or additional recommendations |
|---|---|---|
| Furniture and fittings | Clean with detergent solution, vacuum clean fabric furniture (with high-efficiency filter on exhaust) | Known contaminated and special areas, Cl or Phen |
| Infant incubators | Wash with detergent and dry with disposable wipe | Infected patients or high-risk areas. After cleaning, wipe with Alc or Cl (125 ppm av Cl) |
| Instruments (surgical) | Thermal washer-disinfector followed by steam sterilization if invasive items | Manual clean, followed by steam sterilization if invasive. (Endoscopes—see specific entry above) |
| Laryngoscopes | Heat (sterilization or disinfection) for blade, clean and Alc wipe handle | Clean and immerse blade in Alc 10 min; clean and Alc wipe handle |
| Linen | Machine wash including thermal disinfection | Machine wash including chemical disinfection if thermolabile |
| Locker tops | See furniture and fittings | |
| Mattresses, standard | Water impermeable cover, wash with detergent solution and dry | Disinfect with Cl if contaminated; do not disinfect unnecessarily as this damages the mattress cover |
| Mattresses, pneumatic pressure care | Machine wash including thermal disinfection | Machine wash including chemical disinfection if thermolabile |
| Mops (dry, dust-attracting) | Do not use for more than 2 days without reprocessing or washing | Vacuuming after each use may prolong effective life between processing or washing |
| Mops (wet) | Thermal disinfection in a washing machine then dry: weekly in non-high-risk units and daily in high-risk units (or single-use) | If chemical disinfection is required, rinse in water, soak in Cl (1000 ppm av Cl for 30 min) after use, rinse and store dry |
| Nail brushes (surgical scrub staff hands) | Use only if essential | A sterile nail brush should be used |
| Patient transfer devices: solid (slides and plastic hoists) | Single-patient use in high-risk areas | Clean, then Hyp or Alc |
| Patient transfer devices: fabric (hoists and slings) | Single-patient use in high-risk areas | Machine wash with thermal or chemical disinfection |
| Pillows | Treat as mattresses (standard) | |
| Razors (safety and open) | Single-use or autoclaved | Alc 10 min |
| Razors (electric) | Immerse head in Alc 10 min | |

*continued p. 96*

| Equipment | Routine or preferred method | Acceptable alternative or additional recommendations |
|---|---|---|
| Rooms (terminal cleaning or disinfection) | Non-infected patients: wash surfaces in detergent solution | Infected patients: wash surfaces with detergent solution. Use Cl or Phen if considered necessary |
| Sphygmomanometer cuffs | Single-patient use in high-risk areas or with infected patients | Wash sleeve (with thermal or chemical disinfection) and Alc wipe inflation bladder/tubing |
| Sputum container | Single-use only | |
| Stethoscopes | Wipe head with Alc between patients | With infected patients or in high-risk areas, single-patient use, disinfect with Alc after discharge |
| Suction equipment | Single-use, heat disinfection or sterilization | Clean then Cl |
| Thermometers (oral) | Single-use sleeve | Single-patient use in high-risk areas or infected patient. Clean and Alc for 10 min on patient discharge (include thermometer holder) |
| Thermometers (rectal) | Clean, then Alc for 10 min | |
| Thermometers (electronic clinical) | Single-use sleeve | Single-patient use in high-risk areas or infected patient. Clean, then Alc wipe |
| Thermometers (tympanic) | Single-use sleeve | |
| Toilet seats and flush handles | Wash with detergent and dry | After use by infected patient, or if grossly contaminated, Cl or Phen, rinse and dry |
| Tonometer prisms | Single-use or clean then 500 ppm av Cl for 10 min. Rinse thoroughly | |
| Tooth mugs | Single-patient use | If non-disposable, heat disinfection |
| Toys | Clean first but do not soak soft toys; if contaminated, disinfect by heat (e.g. washing machine) or wiping surface with Alc or Cl | Heavily contaminated soft toys may have to be destroyed |
| Trolley tops (dressings) | (1) Clean with detergent and dry at beginning of dressing round only | (2) If contaminated clean first then use Alc or Cl, Phen and wipe dry |
| Tubing (anaesthetic or ventilator) | Single-use or heat disinfection | |

*continued*

| Equipment | Routine or preferred method | Acceptable alternative or additional recommendations |
|---|---|---|
| Wash basins and taps | Clean with detergent. Use cream cleaner for stains etc. Disinfection not normally required | Disinfection (Cl) may be required if contaminated |
| X-ray equipment | Alc | Clean first if visibly soiled |

# Bibliography

Ayliffe GAJ, Babb JR, Taylor LJ. (1999) *Hospital-Acquired Infection. Principles and Prevention*, 3rd edn. Butterworth Heinemann, Oxford. ISBN: 0750621052.

Ayliffe GAJ, Fraise AP, Geddes AM, Mitchell K, eds. (2000) *Control of Hospital Infection: A Practical Handbook*, 4th edn. Arnold, London. ISBN: 0340759119.

Bennett JV, Brachman PS. (1998) *Hospital Infections*, 4th edn. Little Brown, Boston. ISBN: 0316089028

Block SS, ed. (2001) *Disinfection, Sterilization and Preservation*, 5th edn. Lippincott, Williams & Wilkins, Philadelphia. ISBN: 0683307401.

Collins CH, Kennedy DA. (1999) *Laboratory-Acquired Infections: History, Incidence, Causes and Prevention*, 4th edn. Butterworth Heinemann, Oxford. ISBN: 0750640235.

Damani NN. (2003) *Manual of Infection Control Procedures*, 2nd edn. Greenwich Medical Media, London. ISBN: 1841101079.

Fraise AP, Lambert P, Maillard J-Y, eds. (2003) *Russell, Hugo & Ayliffe's Principles and Practice of Disinfection, Preservation and Sterilization*, 4th edn. Blackwell Science, Oxford. ISBN: 1405101997.

Gardner JF, Peel MM. (1998) *Sterilization, Disinfection and Infection Control*, 3rd edn. Churchill Livingstone, Edinburgh. ISBN: 0443054355.

Hobbs BC, Roberts D. (1993) *Food Poisoning and Food Hygiene*, 6th edn. Arnold, London. ISBN: 034053740.

Lawrence J, May D. (2002) *Infection Control in the Community*. Churchill Livingstone, Edinburgh. ISBN: 0443064067.

Maurer IM. (1985) *Hospital Hygiene*, 3rd edn. Arnold, London. ISBN: 0713144432.

Mayhall CG. (2000) *Hospital Epidemiology and Infection Control*. Lippincott, Williams & Wilkins, Philadelphia. ISBN: 0683306081.

Meers P, McPherson M, Sedgwick J. (1997) *Infection Control in Healthcare*, 2nd edn. Stanley Thornes, Cheltenham. ISBN: 0748733183.

Philpott-Howard J, Casewell M. (1994) *Hospital Infection Control: Policies and Practical Procedures*. Saunders, London. ISBN: 0702016586.

Rutala WA, ed. (1998) *Disinfection, Sterilization and Antisepsis in Healthcare*. Association for Professionals in Infection Control and Epidemiology. Polyscience Publications Inc, Champlain, NY. ISBN: 0921317700.

Wenzel RP, ed. (2003) *Prevention and Control of Nosocomial Infections*, 4th edn. Williams & Wilkins, Baltimore. ISBN: 0781735122.

Wenzel RP, Pittet D, Devaster JM, Butzler JP, Brewer TF, Geddes A, eds. (1998) *A Guide to Infection Control in the Hospital*. BC Decker, Hamilton, Ontario, Canada. ISBN: 1550990593.

Wilson J. (2001) *Infection Control in Clinical Practice*, 2nd edn. Baillière Tindall, London. ISBN: 0702025542.

# Index

Page numbers in *italics* represent figures, those in **bold** represent tables.

absorbent disinfectant granules 74
Advisory Committee in Dangerous
 Pathogens 73
air conditioning systems, *Legionella*
 contamination 32
airway tubes, policy for
 decontamination 93
alcohol 12–13
 babies' incubators 71
 hand disinfection 53
 safety aspects 84
 work benches disinfection 78
alcohol handrubs 53
 *Clostridium difficile* 54
 pathology lab 78
alcoholic formulations
 hygienic hand disinfection 53–54
  pathology lab 78
 irritants 56
 preoperative disinfection of skin 57
 surgical hand disinfection 55
 *see also* alcohol handrubs
aldehydes 15–16
allergy
 antiseptic 55
 latex gloves 57
ampholytic compounds 14
anaesthetic equipment
 disinfection 64–65
 instrument washer-disinfectors
  22
antimicrobial activity, factors
 influencing 3
antiseptic baths, preoperative
 disinfection of skin 57
antiseptics
 allergy to 55
 baths/washbasins 43
 definition 2
 handwashing 51, 53
 prevention of staph colonization in
  neonates 60

Aperlan 11
Approved Codes of Practice to Control
 of Substances Hazardous to
 Health (COSHH) 73
Aquasept 14
aqueous chlorhexidine
 enterococci 31
 mucous membranes disinfection
  58–59
 preoperative disinfection of
  skin 57
aqueous formulations
 hygienic hand disinfection 51–53
 surgical hand disinfection 54–55
aqueous iodine 13
aqueous povidone-iodine
 bacterial spores on skin 58
 mucous membranes disinfection
  58–59
Asep 15
aseptic procedures, alcohol
 handrubs 53
*Aspergillus niger*, disinfectant testing
 88, 89
automated endoscope
 washer-disinfectors 70
 testing/maintenance 70
automated equipment, chemical
 pathology laboratories 77

babies' incubators
 disinfection 71
 policy for decontamination **95**
*bacillus* 27
*Bacillus anthracis* 28
*Bacillus subtilis* 28
bacteria 26
 disinfectant testing 88, 89
bacteria-free water 67
 rinsing 68
bacteria-impermeable filters 64

bacterial spores 27–28
  alcoholic handrub 54
  instrument boilers 24
  on skin 58
bathing/showering, preoperative
    disinfection of skin 57
baths
  cleaning/disinfection 43–44
  decontamination policy 93
bedpans
  effective cleaning 28
  policy for decontamination 93
bedpan washer-disinfectors 23
Betadine 13
black/white fluids 8–9
  safety aspects 85
body fluid spillage,
    cleaning/disinfection 42–43
bovine spongiform encephalopathy
    (BSE) 34
bowls
  cleaning/disinfection 44
  policy for decontamination 94
building maintenance, *Legionella*
    contamination 32–33

calcium hypochlorite 10
*Candida albicans*, disinfectant testing 88,
    89
carpets
  cleaning/disinfection 42
  policy for decontamination 94
catheters, infections 30–31
centrifuges 76–77
Cetavlon 14
chamber washer-disinfectors 22
chemical disinfectants
  body fluid spillage 43
  Control of Substances Hazardous to
    Health (COSHH) 82–83
  discard containers 73
  endoscope disinfection 65
  exposure 81–82
  microbial resistance 27
  post-mortem/mortuary room 78–79
  properties 8–16
  requirements for use in laboratories 73
  safety aspects 80–86
chemical disinfection
  definition 2
  process 3–4
  quality assurance/decontamination
    6–7
  *see also* chemical disinfectants
chemical sterilization, quality
    assurance/decontamination
    5–6

chlorhexidine (diguanides) 12
  prevention of staph colonization in
    neonates 60
  vaginal disinfection 59
  *see also* aqueous chlorhexidine
chlorine 83
  safety aspects 84
chlorine-based disinfectants 9–11
  babies' incubators 71
  body fluid spillage 43
  disinfection policy 19
  enterococci 31
  kitchens 45
  mycobacteria 29
  spillage 74
  toilets/drains 44
  uses/recommended concentrations
    10
  viruses 33
  work benches disinfection 77–78
chlorine dioxide 10
  endoscope 68
  safety aspects 84
Chloros 9
chloroxylenol (para-choro-meta-xylenol;
    PCMX) 9
Cidal 14
Cidex 15
Cidex OPA 15
cleaning
  definition 2
  environmental 40–48
  equipment 45–46
  flexible endoscope 67
  methicillin-resistant *Staph aureus*
    (MRSA) 30
  post-mortem/mortuary room 78
  process 4–5
Clearsol 8
clear soluble phenolics 8
  discard containers 74
  safety aspects 85
  toilets/drains 44
*clostridium* 27
*Clostridium difficile* 27–28
  alcoholic handrub 54
coagulase-negative staphylococci
    30–31
contractors, disinfection policies 17
Control of Substances Hazardous to
    Health (COSHH) 80–82
  Approved Codes of Practice to 73
  chemical disinfectants 82–83
  employers responsibility 80
  future changes 82
  health risks 80
  process 81

cooling towers, cleaning/disinfection 32
costs
  reduction with policies 17
  selection of disinfectant 68
Creutzfeldt-Jakob disease (CJD) 34
  body tissue infectivity 34
  instrumental contamination 34–35
  precautions for cadavers 79
crockery/cutlery, policy for
  decontamination 94
curtains, policy for decontamination **94**
cystoscopes, rigid, heat tolerance 66

decontamination 5–7, **6**
  definition 2
  equipment *see* medical
    equipment/instruments
Diguanides (chlorhexidine) *see*
  chlorhexidine (Diguanides)
dilution 83
dirt, ingrained on skin 58
discard containers 73–74
disinfectant
  bactericidal, requirements 89
  definition 1–2
  fungicidal, requirements 89
  inactivators 87
  quality assurance/decontamination
    5–7, **6**
  user acceptability 56
disinfectant testing 87–91
  aims 87
  CEN standardization 88
  historical background 87–88
  in-use 90
  multiplicity of tests 88
  neutralizers for 88, 90
  organisms 88, 89
  phase I tests (CEN) 88–89
  phase II tests (CEN) 88, 89
  phase III tests (CEN) 88
  reproducibility 87
disinfection
  choice of method 5
  definition 1
  environmental 40–48
  hands *see* handwashing
  principles of 1–2
  process 1–5
disinfection policies 17–20
  choice of disinfectant 19
  formulation 18–19
  organization 17–18
  purpose 17
Diversey detergent sanitizer 10
Domestos 9
drains

cleaning/disinfection 44
  policy for decontamination **94**
dust-attracting mops 45
duvets, policy for decontamination **94**

EN 1040 88
EN 1275 88
EN 13727 89
EN 13624 89
EN 1499 51, 89
EN 1500 51, 54, 89
endoscope(s)
  automated washer-disinfectors 70
  Creutzfeldt-Jakob disease (CJD)
    contamination 35
  disinfectant selection 67–68
  disinfection 65–69, 70
    accessories 70
    cleaning of all channels 65
    difficulties 65
    rinsing 68, 70
  flexible 67
  operative 66–67
  policy for decontamination **94**
  washer-disinfectors *see*
    washer-disinfectors, endoscope
endotracheal tubes, policy for
  decontamination **93**
enterococci 31
*Enterococcus faecium* 31
*Enterococcus hirae*, disinfectant testing 89
*Escherichia coli*, disinfectant testing 89
ethanol *see* alcohol
ethylene oxide
  bacterial spores 27
  operative endoscope 66
  respiratory equipment 64
  sterilization 2
European Committee for
  Standardization (CEN),
  disinfectant testing 88–89

fabrics, cleaning/disinfection 46
faeces, ingrained on skin 58
feeding bottles/teats, policy for
  decontamination **94**
floors
  cleaning/disinfection 40–41
  policy for decontamination **94**
formaldehyde 15
  babies' incubators 71
  room fumigation 75
  safety aspects 84
formalin, room fumigation 75
fumigation, room 75
fumigation, safety cabinet 76
fungal spores 26

fungi 26
  disinfectant testing 88, 89
furniture/fittings, policy for
  decontamination **95**
fusidic acid, *Staphylococcus aureus*
  carriers 59

gas plasma systems
  bacterial spores 27
  sterilization 2
gentamicin, *Staphylococcus aureus*
  carriers 59
Gigasept PA 11
gloves
  body fluid spillage 43
  clean up spillage 74–75
  non-sterile 57
  puncture/contamination 55, 57
  sterile 57
glutaraldehyde 4, 15
  bacterial spores 28
  disinfection policy 19
  endoscope 68
  *Mycobacterium avium-intracellulare* 29
  operative endoscope 66
  safety aspects 84
glycerol, hand disinfection 53
gram-negative bacteria 26
  respiratory equipment contamination
    64
gram-positive bacteria 26

hand disinfection
hygienic 51–54
  surgical 54–55
    alcoholic formulations 55
    aqueous formulations 54–55
  *see also* handwashing
hand disinfection agents
  enterococci 31
  user acceptability 56
  variations 56
hand dryers, hot air 56
hands contamination, pathology lab 78
handwashing 49–56
  cleansing categories **50**
  drying after 56
  pathology lab 78
  routine 51
  technique 52
  user acceptability 56
handwashing agents, disinfectant
  testing (phase 2) 89
hazardous agents, replacement 83
Haz-Tab 10
healthcare applications, thermal
  disinfection 21–24

healthcare laundry 24
heat-sterilized water, rinsing 68
hepatitis A 33
hepatitis B 33
hepatitis C 33
hepatitis viruses 33
hexachlorophane (hexachlorophene)
  13–14
  prevention of staph colonization in
    neonates 60
Hibiscrub 12
Hibitane 12
hospital infection control committee
  17–18
hot air hand dryers 56
hot water tanks, *Legionella pneumophila* 32
humidifiers, disinfection 64
Hycolin 8
hydrogen peroxide 11–12
  safety aspects 84
hypochlorite
  body fluid spillage 43
  check for inactivation 74
  discard containers 74
  safety aspects 85
  testing 90

incubators, babies' *see* babies' incubators
infection outbreaks
  alcohol handrubs 53
  disinfection policy modifications 18
instrument boilers 24
instrument decontamination *see* medical
  equipment/instruments
instrument washer-disinfectors 22
iodine 13
  preoperative disinfection of skin 57
  safety aspects 85
iodophors 13
ionizing radiation sterilization 2
  quality assurance/decontamination 5
irgasan (triclosan) *see* triclosan (irgasan)
isopropanol
  hand disinfection 53
  safety aspects 86
Izal 8

Jeyes fluid 8

Kelsey-Sykes test 87–88
kitchens, cleaning/disinfection 45
Kuru 34

laryngeal mask, policy for
  decontamination **93**
laryngoscopes, policy for
  decontamination **95**

latex gloves, allergy 57
laundry 46–47
 healthcare 24
 UK guidance 46
 viruses 33–34
*legionella* 32–33
*Legionella pneumophila* 32–33
linen, policy for decontamination **95**
Lysol 8

Manusept 14
mattresses
 cleaning/disinfection 44
 policy for decontamination **95**
maximum exposure limit (MEL) 82
medical equipment/instruments 64–72
 decontamination
  policy for **93–97**
  before service/repair 76
 disinfection policy 19
 post-mortem/mortuary room 78
 prion decontamination 34–35
 properties of disinfectant **69**
 surgical instruments *see* surgical
  instruments
methicillin-resistant *Staph aureus*
 (MRSA) 30
microbial resistance
 chemical disinfectants **26**
 thermal disinfectants **26**
microorganisms 26–39
 Control of Substances Hazardous to
  Health (COSHH) 81
 skin colonization 49
Milton 9
mops
 dust-attracting 45
 policy for decontamination **95**
 wet floor 45–46
mortuary room, disinfectants in 78–79
mucous membranes disinfection 49
 preoperative 58–59
mycobacteria 26, 28–29
 disinfectant testing 89
*Mycobacterium avium-intracellulare* 29
*Mycobacterium chelonae* 29
*Mycobacterium fortuitum* 29
*Mycobacterium tuberculosis* 28–29
 operative endoscope 66

nail brushes, policy for decontamination
 **95**
neonate, prevention of staphylococcal
 colonization 60
neutralizers, disinfectant testing 88, 90
Nu-Cidex 11

occupational exposure limit (OEL) 81–82
occupational exposure standard (OES)
 82
operating theaters,
 cleaning/disinfection 40–41
organic matter, effect on disinfectants
 antimicrobial activity 4
orthophthalaldehyde (OPA) 15
 bacterial spores 28
 endoscope 68
 safety aspects 85

paper towels 56
para-choro-meta-xylenol (chloroxylenol;
 PCMX) 9
pathology departments, disinfectants in
 73–79
patient discharge, terminal disinfection
 41
patient transfer devices, policy for
 decontamination **95**
PCMX (para-choro-meta-xylenol;
 chloroxylenol) 9
penicillin, preoperative prophylactic 58
peracetic acid 11
 endoscopes 68
 safety aspects 85
Perasafe 11
Perascope 11
peroxide-based disinfectants 11–12
peroxygen compounds 11–12
 disinfection policy 19
pH, effect on disinfectants antimicrobial
 activity 4
pharmacist, disinfectants 18
phenol, safety aspects 85
'phenol coefficient' 87
phenolics 8–9
 black/white fluids 8–9
  safety aspects 85
 disinfection policy 19
 Enterococci 31
 kitchens 45
 safety aspects 85
 *see also* clear soluble phenolics
pillows, policy for decontamination **95**
plastic aprons, body fluid spillage 43
pneumatic pressure-relieving mattress
 44
 policy for decontamination **95**
post-mortem room, disinfectants in
 78–79
povidone-iodine *see* aqueous
 povidone-iodine
Presept 10
prions 34–35
 cleaning value 2

propan-1-ol, safety aspects 85
propan 2-ol
  disinfectant testing 89
  safety aspects 86
propanol, safety aspects 85
prostheses, infections 30–31
*Pseudomonas aeruginosa*
  disinfectant testing 88, 89
  respiratory equipment contamination
    64

quality assurance 5–7, **6**
quaternary ammonium compounds
  (QACs) 4, 14

razors, policy for decontamination **95**
recontamination, wards/operating
  theaters 40–41
respiratory equipment
  disinfection 64–65
  washer-disinfectors 23
Rideal-Walker test 87
rifampicin, *Staphylococcus aureus* carriers
  59
rigid cystoscopes, heat tolerance 66
risk categories 5
Roccal 14
room fumigation 75
rotavirus, alcoholic handrub 54

safety aspects
  chemical disinfectants 80–86
  individual disinfectants 83–86
safety cabinet fumigation 76
safety data sheet, Control of Substances
    Hazardous to Health (COSHH) 80
Safe working and prevention of
    infection in clinical laboratories
    and similar facilities (2003a) 73
Sanichlor 10
SARS (severe acute respiratory
    syndrome) 33
scrapie 34
severe acute respiratory syndrome
    (SARS) 33
showers, policy for decontamination **93**
skin
  chemical disinfectants 82
  contamination prevention 83
  contamination 49, 83
  disinfectants 2
  disinfection 49
  irritation 56
  preoperative disinfection 57–58
    bacterial spores 58
    longer-term 58

sodium hypochlorite 9–10
  bacterial spores 28
  prions 34
sphygmomanometer cuffs, policy for
    decontamination **96**
spillage 74–75
sporicidal chemical disinfectants,
    bacterial spores 28
sputum container, policy for
    decontamination **96**
staphylococcal colonization, prevention
    in neonates 60
staphylococci, coagulase-negative
    30–31
*Staphylococcus aureus* 29–30
  disinfectant testing 89
  skin colonization 49
  treatment
    nasal carriers 59
    throat carriers 59–60
steam sterilization
  *Bacillus anthracis* 28
  bacterial spores 28
  discard containers 73
  operative endoscope 66
  post-mortem/mortuary room 78
  process 2
  respiratory equipment 64
Stericol 8
sterilant, definition 2
sterile service departments (SSDs) 2–3
sterile service departments, disinfection
    policy 17–18
sterility, definition 1
sterilization
  chemical, quality
    assurance/decontamination
    5–6
  definition 1
  process 1–2
  steam *see* steam sterilization
  thermal, quality
    assurance/decontamination 5
Sterilox 11
Steris 11
Ster-Zac bath concentration 14
  baths/washbasins 43
  prevention of staph colonization in
    neonates 60
Ster-Zac power 13–14
stethoscopes, policy for
    decontamination **96**
suction equipment, policy for
    decontamination **96**
superoxidized water 11
  endoscope 68
surfaces, cleaning/disinfection 40–41

surgical instruments
instrument washer-disinfectors 22
policy for decontamination **95**

Tego 14
temperatures
bedpan/urinal washer-disinfectors
23
thermal disinfection 21–22
time taken **22**
terminal disinfection 41–42
thermal disinfection 21–25
cleaning 2
definition 1
efficacy 21
enterococci 31
health care applications 21–24
kitchens 45
microbial resistance **27**
post-mortem/mortuary room 78
process 3
properties 21
quality assurance/decontamination 7
rigid cystoscopes 66
temperatures 21
thermal sterilization, quality
assurance/decontamination 5
thermometers, policy for
decontamination **96**
tincture of iodine 13
Titan 10
toilets, cleaning/disinfection 44
tonometer prisms, policy for
decontamination **96**
tooth mugs, policy for decontamination
**96**
Totacide 15
toys, policy for decontamination **96**
transmissible spongiform
encephalopathies, cleaning value
2
triclosan (irgasan) 14
baths/washbasins 43
preoperative disinfection of skin 57
Tristel 10

trolley tops, policy for decontamination
**96**
tuberculosis 28–29
respiratory equipment disinfection 65
tubing, policy for decontamination **96**
tunnel washer-disinfectors 22

urinal washer-disinfectors 23

vacuum cleaners 45
vaginal mucosa, disinfection 59
vancomycin-resistant enterococci (VRE)
31
vegetative bacteria 26
ventilator, disinfection 64
Videne 13
Virkon 11–12
viruses 26, 33–34
disinfectant testing 89
enveloped 33
non enveloped 33

wards, cleaning/disinfection 40–41
washbasins
cleaning/disinfection 43–44
policy for decontamination **97**
washer-disinfectors 22–24
automated, endoscope 70
bedpan/urinal 23
endoscope
disinfection 65
testing/maintenance 70
flexible endoscope 67
post-mortem/mortuary room 78
respiratory equipment 23, 64
viruses 33–34
washing bowls
cleaning/disinfection 44
policy for decontamination **94**
work benches disinfection 77–78
workplace exposure limits (WELs) 82

X-ray equipment, policy for
decontamination **97**